AIDS
AND PATIENT
MANAGEMENT:
Legal, Ethical and
Social Issues

AIDS

AND PATIENT MANAGEMENT:
Legal, Ethical and Social Issues

Edited by
Michael D. Witt, Pharm. D., J.D.
Warner & Stackpole

Adapted from the conference
"AIDS—The Ethical, Legal, and Social Considerations,"
sponsored by
Public Responsibility in Medicine and Research (PRIM&R)

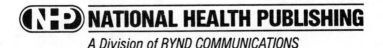

NATIONAL HEALTH PUBLISHING
A Division of RYND COMMUNICATIONS

Copyright © 1986 by
Rynd Communications
99 Painters Mill Road
Owings Mills, MD 21117
(301) 363-6400

Printed in the United States of America
Second Printing
ISBN: 0-932500-46-3
LC: 86-61801

CONTENTS

ACKNOWLEDGMENTS   *ix*

EDITORIAL NOTE   *xi*

    Michael D. Witt, Pharm.D., J.D., Editor

Part I.
Introduction

Acquired Immune Deficiency Syndrome: A Review of Science,
    Health Policy, and Law   3
      Lawrence Gostin, J.D.

Part II.
Public Health Response to the AIDS Crisis

Addressing Public Health Concerns of the City of San Francisco   27
    Mervyn Silverman, M.D.

Government Involvement and the Development of Public Policy
    in AIDS Research and Reporting   36
      Edward N. Brandt, Jr., M.D., Ph.D.

Balancing Individual and Societal Rights   44
    Sheldon Landesman, M.D.

Part III.
The Complications of AIDS Research

Placebo-Controlled, Double-Blind Research on Patients with AIDS   51
    Martin S. Hirsch, M.D.

Controlled Therapeutic Trials on Patients with AIDS   53
    Clyde Crumpacker, M.D.

Protection of Personal Rights   60
    Jeffrey Levi

Ethical and Moral Issues in AIDS Research   64
    Jerome E. Groopman, M.D.

The Effects of Discrimination Against Gays 65
Michael Callen

Confidentiality and AIDS Research: Where Research and Personal
Rights Conflict 69
Carol Levine, M.A.

Appendix: Guidelines for Confidentiality in Research on AIDS 72
Ronald Bayer, Carol Levine, and Thomas H. Murray

Part IV.
Legal Problems of AIDS Patients and Health Care Providers

Legal Implications of the AIDS Epidemic 89
Leonard Glantz, J.D.

The Rights of Patients Hospitalized with AIDS 90
George J. Annas, J.D., M.P.H.

Quarantine and AIDS 93
Alvin Novick, M.D.

Disability and Estate Planning Considerations 96
Steven Ansolabehere, J.D.

The Right to Receive Health Care 100
Michael Callen

Appendix: Connecticut Quarantine Statute 106
Connecticut Public Act. No. 84-336

Part V.
The Impact of AIDS on the Patient,
Family, Friends, and Community

Psychiatric Illness in Patients with AIDS 113
Joseph Barbuto, M.D.

Mental Health Needs of People with AIDS 117
Marshall Forstein, M.D.

To Have Without Holding: Memories of Life with a Person with AIDS 121
Joseph Interrante, Ph.D.

Social Impact on Dating in the Gay Community 125
David McWhirter, M.D.

Social Support Services: AIDS Action Committees 127
Lawrence Kessler

Part VI.
HTLV-III Screening and the Blood Supply

Public Health Policies and Concerns   135
  Kenneth Mayer, M.D.

Critical Blood Banking Issues   140
  Peter Page, M.D.

The Gift of Blood: Social Policy in Evolution   150
  Johanna Pindyck, M.D.

Research Risks and Federally-Funded Studies   154
  F. William Dommel, Jr.

Part VII.
Cultural and Historical Perspectives

Historical Analogies to the AIDS Epidemic   159
  Allan M. Brandt, Ph.D.

Public Health and Social Disease   164
  Barbara G. Rosenkrantz, Ph.D.

Global Distribution of AIDS   166
  Sheldon Landesman, M.D.

Part VIII.
Issues in Social Science Research

Social Research on AIDS   173
  Joan Sieber, Ph.D.

Anxiety and Informed Consent   176
  Barbara Stanley, Ph.D.

Sociomedical Research Priorities in AIDS   177
  John L. Martin, Ph.D., M.P.H.

Issues in AIDS Epidemiology   181
  William M. Hamilton, Ph.D.

Appendix: Ethical Issues in Psychological Research on AIDS   185
  American Psychological Association

Part IX.
Guidelines for the Management of AIDS Patients

The Case Definition of AIDS   195
  Centers for Disease Control

Recommendations for Preventing Transmission of Infection with Human
   T-Lymphotrophic Virus Type III/Lymphadenopathy-Associated
   Virus in the Workplace   200
    Centers for Disease Control

Acquired Immune Deficiency Syndrome (AIDS): Precautions
   for Clinical and Laboratory Staffs   214
    Centers for Disease Control

Acquired Immunodeficiency Syndrome (AIDS): Precautions
   for Health-Care Workers and Allied Professionals   218
    Centers for Disease Control

Recommendations for Preventing Possible Transmission of Human
   T-Lymphotrophic Virus Type III/Lymphadenopathy-Associated
   Virus from Tears   220
    Centers for Disease Control

Cleaning, Disinfection, and Sterilization of Hospital Equipment   223
    Centers for Disease Control

General Infection Control Guidelines for Pre-hospital
   Care Personnel   234
    Massachusetts Department of Public Health
    Office of Emergency Medical Services

Cleaning Procedures for Ambulance Equipment and Interior   235
    Massachusetts Department of Public Health
    Office of Emergency Medical Services

Infection Control Guidelines for Handling Blood Products   237
    Visiting Nurse Association of Boston

Care of AIDS Patient in Home Setting   239
    Visiting Nurse Association of Boston

A Hospitalwide Approach to AIDS   240
    Patricia Navicky, R.N.
    Lemuel Shattuck Hospital

ABOUT THE EDITOR   253

INDEX   255

ACKNOWLEDGMENTS

Many people were instrumental in making the publication of these proceedings a reality. I mention a few of these professionals below and thank them for their contributions.

The participants in the conference reviewed and assisted greatly in the process of creating a document from a series of presentations. This task is always an arduous one. The sponsors of the conference, Tufts University School of Medicine and PRIM&R, are recognized also for their efforts.

I thank the experts at Rynd Communications for reviewing the manuscript, making helpful suggestions, and exercising considerable patience in each phase of document production. It is amazing to me how few people understand the value of a quality publishing company. They are capable of making a project such as this a delight.

The partners at Warner and Stackpole allowed me to utilize the full (and considerable) resources of the law firm to prepare this manuscript. Their understanding, patience, and support for me, my ideas, and my projects is recognized with gratitude. I thank Alan H. Einhorn, Chairman of the Health Care Department at Warner and Stackpole, for sharing his expertise and knowledge about the AIDS pandemic and for critically reviewing the manuscript.

I thank Beth L. Secrest, my secretary, for her perserverance, professionalism, and active participation in this project. Further, I recognize the considerable contribution of Heather E. Jenkins, Carolyn M. Anderson, and Helen B. Long of the firm's Word Processing Department. Brian J. Harkins, J.D. provided essential research and technical support.

My wife, Teresa Goggins Witt, reviewed and edited numerous drafts of the manuscript and made many useful suggestions for revisions. Her assistance is very much appreciated.

Finally, many physicians and scientists have responded to the AIDS crisis in an admirable, selfless manner. Despite serious personal risk, physicians and nurses treat infected individuals to the limits of their abilities with compassion and respect. Microbiologists and infectious disease specialists, working with the various strains of the HTLV-III virus, risk infection and death. I share the hope of many people that these courageous researchers are able to effect a cure for this dread disease. These persons deserve our sincere thanks.

It seems almost ironic, however, that public, professional, and government pressure on organized medicine is so great at a time when deficit budgeteers systematically dismantle the medical–industrial complex that will in time develop a treatment for AIDS. It remains to be seen whether the medical establishment will be able to react in similar fashion to the next crisis, especially in light of the growing trend of many professionals to leave medicine because of increasingly burdensome regulatory and other administrative constraints on helping sick people to become well.

EDITORIAL NOTE

The lectures that formed the basis for this book were presented at a conference entitled "AIDS: The Ethical, Legal and Social Considerations." The conference was sponsored jointly by Tufts New England Medical Center and Public Responsibility in Medicine and Research (PRIM&R). The faculty included luminaries from around the country, most of whom have been directly involved in combating the AIDS epidemic since it first appeared in the United States in 1981.

Although the conference was held on April 24–25, 1985, this book is not a static record of the state of AIDS information available on those dates. As I began editing, I found that the time needed to edit the conference transcripts would be in constant conflict with the rapidly growing body of knowledge about AIDS. To keep this book from becoming a historical document immediately upon its publication, I felt that it was important to revise the transcripts to present current information. Many of the numerical estimates of mortality and morbidity, treatment, and testing issues have been altered to reflect the present opinions of the participants. Where appropriate, concepts considered to be useful and correct at the time of the conference were reconsidered and revised to reflect additional experiences of the participants. With this perspective in mind, the book not only represents a snapshot of the thoughts, biases, and perspectives of the participants at the time, but also incorporates the revised thinking of the participants and the editor.

As you will see, this faculty included not only public health officers, epidemiologists, infectious disease experts, virologists, microbiologists, psychiatrists, and other medical scientists, but also included attorneys, ethicists, gay rights proponents, historians, social scientists and lay people who have experienced the disease themselves. Together they offer an amalgam of unique perspectives that summarizes how the world views the AIDS epidemic. Some of the articles would have a definite place in scholarly journals or monographs. Others would not conform to strict academic standards but have been included because they yield information that is rich in intense emotion and insight. There are presentations of scientific data that are both stirring and insightful. There are also accounts of personal experiences with AIDS that are so heartrending as to make the reader actually feel the pain and suffering that this disease has caused. I cannot say that I was in concord with each lecturer; however, no matter how biased I may have found an individual's perspective, I took great care to leave his or her language intact for your consideration.

As an aside, I felt that the faculty did not adequately address the issues relating to intravenous drug use and transmission of AIDS. The oversight appears to reflect the involvement of many of the faculty members in the problem of AIDS in the gay community. Given what is now known about intravenous drug abuse and AIDS, I believe that if the conference were held again, more serious attention would be given to the problem.

The reader will find that this book has been supplemented with contributions unrelated to the conference. In a book that presented such a diverse set of medical and legal viewpoints, it seemed important to include an introduction that tied them all together in a coherent overview of "science, health policy, and law." I took the liberty of asking Larry Gostin, a fine attorney and academician at the Harvard School of Public Health (also the new Executive Director of the American Society of Law and Medicine), to prepare that introduction. He has done an admirable job. Also, I have included materials from the Centers for Disease Control and several Boston-area health care facilities in Part IX for your use.

At the very least, this book summarizes most of the scientific and human issues we have been struggling with. At most, the book creates a template for other people to use when they desire a thorough airing of complex scientific and policy issues. I hope that you find it to be useful and informative.

Michael D. Witt
Boston, Massachusetts
February 24, 1986

PART I
Introduction

Acquired Immune Deficiency Syndrome:
A Review of Science, Health Policy, and Law

Lawrence Gostin, J.D.*
Senior Research Fellow, Faculty of Public Health
Harvard University

Acquired immune deficiency syndrome (AIDS) poses the greatest threat to public health of any communicable disease in contemporary times; the effort to reduce its spread is the U.S. government's top health priority.[1] It is unique in its combination of risk factors: the underlying disease process cannot currently be prevented or treated; the etiologic viral agent is noted for its propensity to exhibit phenotypic variability and to mutate easily, making the future development of vaccines or treatment more difficult; there is no finite incubation period, so carriers of the virus are chronically infectious; and, the major risk groups each are vulnerable to social prejudice and private discrimination, posing special problems for public health officials seeking to identify persons carrying the virus and capable of transmitting it. Public concern is rife and could itself be viewed as a secondary social epidemic of panic. AIDS therefore poses an incomparable challenge for health policymakers who must seek methods of reducing the spread of the disease and to help ensure the public safety consistent with the protection of individual respect and autonomy.

It is necessary first to set out the medical and epidemiologic data so that policy accurately follows scientific knowledge of the communication of the disease. Any other course would allow the secondary social epidemic of fear and misinformation to restrict individual autonomy and discriminate against insular populations without any measurable impact on the public health. After reviewing the scientific literature relating to the etiology and transmission of AIDS, there will be an analysis of the major public policy options available to public health officials and legislators.

Scientific Data

AIDS: A Case Definition

AIDS was first identified in the United States in 1981 with the reporting of cases of five gay men who died from an unusual lung infection due to a protozoan

*Professor William Curran and the author have a sole source contract with the U.S. Department of Health and Human Services to review health policy and law relating to the AIDS epidemic. Both Professor Curran and Mr. Gostin are attorneys associated with the law firm of Warner and Stackpole in Boston. A fuller report of their final results will be published elsewhere. The author would like to thank Mary Clarke for her research efforts in this national AIDS project.

parasite, Pneumocystis carinii; others had a rare neoplasm, Kaposi's sarcoma.[2] Similar cases were reported thereafter.[3] In all of the cases the infections or cancer were opportunistic in that they occur only in those who are immunosuppressed. There was a lack of T-4 lymphocytes or white blood cells (which are "helper" or regulatory cells) necessary for the immune response. In each reported case, the patient was previously healthy, leading to the conclusion that the attacks on their immune systems had been acquired. As the immunosuppressed patients manifested one or more forms of disease, it was called a syndrome. The Centers for Disease Control (CDC) termed it acquired immunodeficiency syndrome.

The CDC developed a case definition of AIDS for national reporting purposes in 1982[4] which was endorsed by the World Health Organization for use in countries where appropriate technologies are available:[5] a reliably diagnosed disease[6] which is at least moderately indicative of an underlying cellular immunodeficiency[7] when no known cause for reduced resistance to that disease is present.[8] AIDS was originally defined before its etiology was known. Current laboratory tests for AIDS-related antibodies make it possible to include additional serious conditions in the syndrome where the patient is seropositive.[9]

AIDS: A Clinical Spectrum

The surveillance definition of AIDS was developed for precision, consistency in interpretation, and specificity in order to provide useful data on disease trends. The CDC definition is only a narrow point on a wide spectrum of illness which is still not fully understood.[10,11] The great majority of people infected with the AIDS related virus are asymptomatic. The virus is known also to cause an acute, transient nonspecific syndrome. It is a mononucleosis-type illness characterized by lymphadenopathy (a disease process affecting the lymph nodes), prolonged unexplained fever, myalgia (muscular pain), fatigue or lethargy, gastrointestinal symptoms, sore throat, and diarrhea. This acute AIDS-related syndrome is not directly life-threatening, although a fraction of cases will advance into more serious symptoms.

AIDS-related complex (ARC) is a more serious level of AIDS-related infection. The range of manifestations is wide, including a variety of opportunistic infections, several types of malignancy and neurologic disorders. The latter is particularly important in a legal study as it can affect the person's competency and behavior patterns. It is estimated that in some 30%–60% of cases of AIDS-related infection there is an observable impact on the central nervous system leading to symptoms of dementia.[12]

AIDS, then, should be viewed as a continuum of disease manifestations. The phenomenon is so recent that science does not yet have a full understanding of the natural history of the disease; the potential long-term sequelae among persons exposed to the virus is chilling. Current studies are designed to discover the process and time periods involved for infective asymptomatic persons to develop acute lymphadenopathy syndrome, ARC, and then "frank" AIDS. Information to date is worrying. In six different studies, the proportion of seropositive persons in whom "frank" AIDS developed during follow-up periods of one to five years ranged from 4%–19%. In several of those studies signs of acute AIDS-related symptoms have developed in up to an additional 25% of those exposed to the virus.

The occurrence of AIDS in previously healthy young people suggests that the AIDS-related virus may be sufficient to cause the disease. But there are theories that point to cofactors which may be involved in the disease process. The demonstrated greater susceptibility of infants to the AIDS-related virus may result from the immaturity of the neonatal immune system.[13] It is possible, but not yet demonstrated, that other factors which suppress the immune system may modify the disease process. Such factors could include the medical use of steroids or antineoplastic agents, other coexisting immunosuppressant diseases, severe protein-calorie malnutrition, or even old age. Similar unconfirmed hypotheses have focused on a specific or nonspecific "overload" of the immune system impairing its function in vulnerable patients.

Whatever the disease process may turn out to be, for public health purposes it should be assumed that those who are infected with the AIDS-related virus are capable of communicating the infection. It does not matter whether the individual is asymptomatic or manifesting the symptoms of ARC or frank AIDS. A legal policy analysis cannot logically differentiate among those who harbor the virus and can transmit it.

AIDS: The Epidemic

The epidemiologic evidence of AIDS-related infection is sobering. There have been more than 20,000 CDC-defined cases reported; more than half have been reported during the preceding 12 months. The case fatality rate is over 50% in total and over 75% for patients diagnosed before January 1983. There are well documented risk groups for the disease. Approximately 73% of the total number of reported AIDS cases are gay or bisexual men (12% also use intravenous drugs); 17% are heterosexual men or women who use intravenous drugs; 1.5% with no other risk factor have received a transfusion of whole blood or one of its components within five years of the diagnosis; and 0.7% are persons with hemophilia who had received clotting factor concentrates. There are 1% who are heterosexual partners of persons with increased risk of AIDS who are not themselves in a risk group. The remaining 6.4% are not classifiable by recognized risk factors, but some half of these people were born outside of the United States in countries, mostly Haiti, where many AIDS cases have not been associated with known risk factors. Of the 200 or more diagnosed infants and children, almost all were born to a parent in an identified risk category. It is clear, therefore, that membership within certain population groups greatly increases the chance of contracting the disease.

For every person who has the CDC definition of AIDS, there are between 50 and 100 who have the infection. If the infection-to-AIDS ratio is correct, then one to two million people in the United States have been infected with the virus. Moreover, predictive models indicate that over 12,000 additional cases of AIDS will be reported by July 1986 with chilling implications for the number of people estimated to be infected.[14]

This geometric increase in the number of predicted potential carriers of the virus has charged the atmosphere of health policy debate. Others have given more cautious estimates of increased prevalence of the virus and the disease, suggesting that the curve will flatten out due to a saturation of the risk groups;[15] these commentators note that there has been a relatively steady 1% of the population of AIDS cases which are outside known risk groups, indicating that the disease may not move to nonrisk groups as has occurred in other countries. There are currently no reliable indicators as to whether the acceleration or saturation theory is correct. In any case, public health measures must of necessity focus on those populations at greatest risk—both for the sake of individuals within those populations and for the wider community. On one level, intensive public health measures seem to discriminate and further stigmatize these populations. But this analysis does those groups a disservice—first, by falsely assuming that there is some shame or fault to be associated with one of these groups and, second, to take less care in preventing the spread of disease within these groups than would be taken for infectious diseases in any other context. This is not to suggest that confidentiality and autonomy of these groups are not important. The assumption of this introduction, however, is that policy in relation to AIDS should, as with any other disease, reflect the scientific facts concerning its infectiousness, and should use all reasonable measures necessary to reduce its spread.

AIDS Related Virus: Antibody Testing

It is rare for the etiologic agent of a disease to be isolated quickly after the discovery of the disease. However, because of the urgent need to understand AIDS, its probable cause was discovered in late 1983. It is a retrovirus variously termed human T-cell lymphotropic (leukemia) virus type III (HTLV-III),[16,17] lymphadenopathy-associated virus (LAV)[18,19] or AIDS-related virus (ARV).[20] All three are probably the same agent.[21] In order to avoid confusion, new terminology was recently proposed—human immunodeficiency virus (HIV). Retrovirus infections in animals persist for long periods, usually for life. The AIDS-related virus has been shown to persist in humans for many years; until otherwise demonstrated, it must be assumed that once infected with the virus a person is chronically infectious.

An enzyme-linked immunosorbent assay (ELISA) has been developed to detect antibodies to the AIDS-related virus.[22] A reactive result indicates that the person has been exposed to the virus and has mounted an immunologic response (serum antibodies). However, the test is not an antigen test and a positive result does not necessarily mean that the person currently harbors the virus.

The ELISA test has been shown to be reasonably "sensitive" by registering positive in a high proportion of patients with AIDS; and reasonably "specific" by registering positive in a low proportion of healthy volunteer blood donors. Excluding borderline results, the range of sensitivity of the test has been shown to be 93.4%–99.6% and the range of specificity 98.6%–99.6%.[22-25] Seroepidemiologic studies within each of the major risk groups,[20] including hemophilia patients,[26-29] gay men[30] and parenteral drug users,[30] shows uniformly high rates of positivity, while positivity among heterosexual men and women who are not members of known risk groups is extremely low.[21-23]

Despite the sensitivity and specificity of the test, the significance of a positive result is unclear. Reactive tests may be due to subclinical infection, to immunity, to an active carrier state or may represent false-positive reactions such as crossreactivity to antigens or other viruses.[22] False-positives occur where the test shows an immunologic response to HTLV-III when in fact there is no such response. The rate of false-positives probably depends upon the prevalence of antibody in the donor population, with higher prevalence resulting in more meaningful test results.[23] The range of false-positive rates is estimated to be between 0.17%–0.89% of the total population tested. But out of every hundred persons who are tested positive, anywhere from one-half to over two-thirds may be false-positives.[23,24]

To confirm whether a positive test is a true-positive a confirmatory ELISA test can be given. In one study from 131 blood banks and centers, less than one-third of the initially reactive blood units were repeatedly reactive.[31] A second ELISA test can reduce false-positives, but not eliminate them.[32] A more expensive ($100, compared with $2-$3) and technically more difficult confirmatory test, the Western blot, can be performed. This test identifies antibodies and proteins of a specific molecular weight.[33] Another confirmatory test is the immunofluorescence assay (IFA).

AIDS Related Virus: Transmissability

It is theoretically possible for the AIDS-related virus to be found in any body fluid which contains lymphocytes. Scientists have successfully isolated and cultured live viruses from the blood,[34] semen,[34,35] saliva,[36] tears[37], and vaginal secretions of patients with AIDS, AIDS-related symptoms, or infected asymptomatic individuals. Other body fluids that might potentially harbor the live virus are breast milk, urine, and feces. Live viruses can transmit disease, but the presence of a live virus in low concentrations in a body fluid is not necessarily significant. The AIDS-related virus is quite difficult to communicate; it requires a direct transfer of body fluid through intimate physical contact. Almost all cases of transfer in the United States have occurred through one or more of four routes:[14] sexual contact, intravenous drug administration with contaminated needles, transfusion of blood and blood products, and passage of the virus from infected mothers to their newborns. Epidemiologic studies have identified specific behavioral risk factors such as increased number of sexual partners and receptive anal intercourse or practices associated with rectal trauma. The acquisition of the virus by heterosexual contact has been well-documented.[38,39,42] Male to female transmission is thought to be more efficient and is epidemiologically significant in the United States. Female to male transmission is reported from central Africa;[40,41] there is some tentative confirmatory evidence in the United States[38] which emphasizes the role of female prostitutes in this form of transmission.

The AIDS-related virus is quite fragile. There is increasing evidence that it is not transmitted through casual contact. Studies showing the extreme rarity with which infection is transmitted from prolonged and close household contact illustrate that mere exposure to and touching of infected persons does not pose a real risk of virus transmission.[42,43]

Public Policy

The overriding public policy objective of health law is to prevent serious harm. Compulsory measures are justified where they are clearly necessary to impede the spread of infectious disease, and where interference with liberty, autonomy or privacy is not disproportionate to the health benefit to be achieved.

The classic public health response to highly infectious disease requires three steps. First, identify those who harbor the virus either by focusing on patients manifesting the disease or through testing and screening of populations at risk. Second, report infectious individuals to public health officials who keep a register. Third, isolate those capable of transmitting the infection. This traditional model is unsuited to the AIDS epidemic. The AIDS-related virus is not confined to any discrete geographic area or population; if control measures applied to all carriers of the virus, they could affect a million or more human beings. The virus is not incubated for a short period and cannot be prevented or treated. Accordingly, any compulsory measure would have to persist indefinitely, potentially for life, as persons would continually be capable of transmitting the virus. Any measures designed to exclude individuals from society, or any part of society such as schools, would be unnecessarily restrictive of liberty, as the virus is not transmitted when infected individuals are socially integrated with other people; exclusion of AIDS carriers from society would be ineffective in controlling the spread of the disease while denying them even a rudimentary opportunity for a normal integrated life. Compulsory measures which rely on controlling the private and intimate behavior involved in the most efficient modes of transmission would have to overcome such insuperable barriers as identifying all those who could transmit the disease, predicting their future behavior, and controlling that behavior. Social science does not even begin to have the tools to accomplish these objectives, and any compulsory measures could well have the reverse effect by reducing compliance with voluntary efforts and providing a major disincentive to seek testing, counselling and treatment.

Experience with highly analogous diseases such as hepatitis B has demonstrated that voluntary compliance can reduce the spread of the disease;[43] emerging evidence on AIDS already shows significant alteration of behavior necessary to reduce spread within risk groups.[44] Further, experience with the use of compulsory measures in analogous diseases such as venereal diseases shows them to be ineffective, discriminatory, and invidious.[45,46] In the absence of historical or contemporary evidence that compulsory measures do change behavior more effectively than voluntary programs based upon focused public education and counseling,[47] and given the evidence of broad voluntary behavior change in groups at risk for AIDS, there is no rational basis for the introduction of coercive measures.

It is the assumption of this introduction, therefore, that when the adverse effects on liberty, autonomy, privacy, and social respect and integrity of affected individuals and groups are wholly disproportionate to the uncertain benefit to public health, then compulsory measures are unjustified.

It is perhaps understandable that many members of the public choose a different formula for risk management than adopted in this introduction. A parent of a school child might argue that *any* potentially lethal risk is unacceptable if it is preventable through the use of compulsory measures, *e.g.*, excluding children or adults harboring the virus from ordinary life. So long as medical researchers are unable entirely to exclude the probability of casual transfer of the virus, some argue it is best to err on the side of caution. Negligible risks, however, are part of ordinary life and small risks are fully accepted in society. Any social activity entails some small risk—even going to school in a motor vehicle or as a pedestrian. So long as those risks are negligible compared with the benefits of social and human discourse, we accept them. It is hardly asking too much to accept the most remote possibility of communication of the virus given the benefits of allowing individuals to live freely in their communities. It would be otherwise if the health risks they posed were real, and the use of public health powers were effective.

The use of compulsory powers represents a certain restriction of individual liberty and autonomy for many. If we take individual freedom seriously, this certain deprivation is simply too great a price to pay in exchange for a negligible and theoretical impact on public health.

There follows an analysis of classic public health powers as they could potentially apply to AIDS, showing what policies have already been adopted and those that could be adopted.

Screening

The degree of overall reliability and the safeguards required when screening blood for the AIDS-related antibody depends upon the use to be made of the results. Where the results of the screening are applied or evaluated in the aggregate and there is no impact on any individual person, the ELISA alone may often be sufficient in light of its high sensitivity and specificity. The ELISA test, in the absence of any inexpensive, more reliable procedure, can be invaluable for helping ensure the safety of the blood supply or for research purposes.[22]

Where disclosure of results has the potential to adversely affect the individual through social prejudice and discrimination, or where it is used as a condition precedent to compulsory powers, then the need for reliability and attendent safeguards becomes much greater. In cases where the general health benefit to be achieved by the screening is clearly outweighed by the potential for adverse social and legal consequences for the individual, screening should not take place at all. Save for the use of screening the blood supply, screening donations to sperm banks, and for research purposes, there is no convincing public health rationale for any adventure into testing and screening the various potential populations examined below. There are three overriding reasons for this conclusion. First, there is an unacceptably high false-positive rate. Potentially, out of every 100 individuals in a sample of healthy blood donors found to be seropositive on an initial ELISA test, 20 will be repeatedly reactive and only four will be Western blot positive.[24] If screening were to result in any adverse consequences for individuals, these consequences would be visited upon an unacceptably high number of people without sufficient justification that they harbor the virus. Second, even if a more reliable antigen test were developed for AIDS, the question arises as to what would be done with the information obtained from the screening. Clearly the individual would be informed and would be given sufficient information and counseling necessary to allow that person willingly to change behavior. However, individuals predisposed to such behavior changes currently can voluntarily seek the test at alternative test sites. Compulsory measures could be used which interfered with the person's liberty (*e.g.*, quarantine), autonomy (*e.g.*, exclusion from school or job) or privacy (*e.g.*, contact tracing). But this would have the almost certain result of making people in risk groups much more reluctant to seek testing and treatment, and would severely reduce compliance with voluntary public health measures. Further, the mere holding of highly sensitive information poses special ethical and legal quandaries. A seropositive status potentially makes that individual a risk to others. Does this entail a duty to warn those most at risk? A legal duty to warn those who are in foreseeable danger has already been superimposed upon confidential therapist–patient relationships;[48] it is not inconceivable that warning spouses or known sexual partners or advising public health officials would be judicially required in some jurisdictions.

A third reason not to introduce universal screening is, as already discussed, the sheer numbers of people involved. This disadvantage might not apply to more limited screening such as for prehospital admission, for prenatal and premarital testing, or for health care workers. Yet to single out any of these groups from all the many others who carry the virus requires a strong justification, such as the special high risk involved with the group and/or the availability of clear measures to make use of the information for preventitive purposes. As will be seen below, it is difficult to find any such compelling justifications for screening any particular population on the scientific and epidemiologic evidence currently available.

There are a great many possibilities for screening of particular populations that could be considered. Screening programs might focus on populations which might have higher incidences of the virus such as the major risk groups, at drug treatment centers, in certain geographic areas; or higher than average risk settings for the transfer of the virus such as hospitals or emergency rooms, dental or optician services; vulnerability of the population, such as with school children; or even economic factors, such as for insurance purposes.

A coherent analysis of each of these areas would be too lengthy to include here. But, a few of the more discussed screening possibilities are briefly reviewed below.

Blood Donors. FDA recommendations provide for screening of all plasma and blood for HTLV-III antibodies: (1) reactive units should not be transfused; (2) the blood donor should be notified only upon a positive result from a second ELISA or other test; (3) such a donor should be referred to a physician for evaluation; and, (4) positive test results should be kept confidential.[49] This policy represents a prudent course given the absolute importance of protecting the blood supply. To discard blood, even on the basis of a single reactive test, would not infringe on the autonomy of any individual nor should it serve as a disincentive to donate blood. Placing the names of individuals on a blood referral registry requires strict confidentiality. Disclosure would be likely to result in social prejudice and discrimination.

Major blood banks have developed effective systems of confidentiality. They have a duty of confidentiality which is implied by the relationship they form with donors. Such a duty can be enforced in some states by statute; in the absence of statute there is a common law remedy for breach of confidentiality.[50] As the common law remedy is ancient and unsure there is a case for the enactment of statutory protections of confidentiality in jurisdictions where there are none. The federal government has already intervened to require regulation of confidentiality in the analogous context of addiction, alcoholism and detoxification records.[51] An extension of these regulations would be useful to consider in relation to blood donations.[52] Ensuring the confidentiality of donors would remove any possible disincentive to giving blood and would extend significant protection in safeguarding the privacy of donors.

One problem remains and that is the reach of judicial process. As there is no formal privilege between donor and blood bank, a litigant conceivably could subpoena the records of blood donors.[53] A case is pending before the Supreme Court of Florida where a donee who developed AIDS is seeking such records.[54] Blood banks often do hold the information necessary to trace donations of blood to specific recipients, even many years after the fact.

Prehospital Admission and Health Care Workers. Hospital settings pose special risks in the communication of any disease, particularly AIDS-related infections. The source of the infection could rest either with the patient or the health care worker. Potential transfer of body fluids in minute amounts could occur through contact with cuts, open sores, needle stick accidents and the like. Surgery poses one of the most obvious risk factors.

It is because of the possibility of communication in the hospital setting that proposals for special screening procedures for patients and/or for health care workers could be considered. A further possible reason for such screening is to clarify hospital liability issues. If a patient were to seroconvert or develop signs of AIDS following a period of hospital care, knowing that person's serologic status prior to admission would clarify liability issues.

Screening of any kind is fraught with difficulties, as examined above. But these difficulties can be overcome if there is clear evidence of special risk and the availability of effective measures to reduce the spread of infection. Neither justification is currently available for screening of patients or health care workers. Studies show that hospital and laboratory settings do not pose significant risk of transfer of the AIDS-related virus.[55,56] The major areas of concern to date have been needle stick accidents. The evidence shows that HTLV-III transmission from an isolated parenteral response is low. Health care workers also do not appear to have contracted the virus from contact with patients from other causes such as cuts, open wounds or attending to sanitary needs of patients, although future occurrences cannot be ruled out. Special attention should be given to risks taken during surgery by surgeons as well as patients.

Control measures in hospital settings to reduce the spread of the virus are at present unnecessary. Exclusion of a seropositive patient from admission to hospital would be wrong both legally and ethically; the hospital has a duty to treat those presenting with a genuine medical condition. Dismissal of a surgeon or other health care worker who is seropositive would have to be based upon clear evidence that he or she poses a danger of infecting others. Knowing that a person carries the AIDS-related virus might well result in greater attention to preventive measures such as protecting open sores from exposure to a patient's blood. Nevertheless such precautions should be taken by prudent professionals. In the absence of clear evidence of special risks of communication and given the myriad problems associated with screening, uniform testing of all patients or health care workers is not justified.

U.S. government guidelines set out precautions for clinical aı.J laboratory staffs which include advice on avoiding accidental wounds from sharp instruments contaminated with potentially infectious material and avoiding contact of open lesions with material from patients.[57] Further guidelines have been published for precautions for health care workers and allied professionals such as dental care personnel and morticians.[58] These guidelines do not resort to screening or compulsory measures.

Premarital and Prenatal Screening. As one of the specific risk groups for AIDS-related infection is infants who contract the virus from their mothers in utero, during childbirth or postnatally, one obvious target for screening could be women who may bear children. Such screening could take place as a condition precedent to the acquisition of a marriage license or as part of the prenatal care of women. The obvious benefit of this screening is that it could provide a focus for counseling; any mother who tests positive would be advised not to bear children. It might conceivably be used by extremists as an opportunity for more repressive measures such as sterilization of carriers of the AIDS-related virus.

Preventing women who harbor the virus from having children clearly would reduce, even if to a very small degree, the spread of the disease. Yet, there is insufficient evidence to justify such large scale mandatory screening procedures. Perinatal transmission of the virus is still not a major cause of spread of the disease. Less intrusive measures still can be used to seek to reduce this form of transmission. Those women in risk groups can, and should, be advised of the possibility of transferring the virus to infants; this represents the view of the Public Health Service. These women should have the opportunity to be tested for HTLV-III antibodies and to receive full information and counseling. This should prove to cover most women who might transfer the virus to their babies. It would be premature to test all women at the time of marriage or prenatally given the number of false-positives the test would produce and the resultant stress and expense.

Control Measures

Public health measures are predicated not only upon identifying individuals capable of transmitting infection but also upon taking positive action against those harboring a potentially lethal virus to prevent its spread. Voluntary measures should always be used as long as they are reasonably effective and there are no compulsory powers which would have a more significant impact on reducing the spread of the virus. At present almost all American jurisdictions rely solely on voluntary efforts such as informing those who test positive for HTVL-III antibodies of the risks of transmission, providing individual counseling and public education. These individual and public education measures clearly have altered behavior, which is evidenced by the profound reduction in the number of cases of rectal gonorrhea in the gay community.

Health policy options, however, extend beyond voluntary efforts. The state has a right to exercise its police powers for the public welfare. Under the principle of "necessity," "a community has the right to protect itself against an epidemic of disease which threatens the safety of its members."[59] Among the control measures typically provided for in state public health statutes are compulsory examination and treatment including immunization, disinfection, reporting and registering, and quarantine. As AIDS is a disease which has no prevention or treatment, the only forms of potentially effective control available under public health statutes are reporting, registering, and quarantine. Our group at Harvard is under a sole source contract with the U.S. Department of Health and Human Services which will, *inter alia*, examine state statutes to determine whether they would be construed to apply to AIDS. It is the intention here to discuss whether the courts would be likely to uphold as constitutional compulsory public health powers designed to prevent the spread of AIDS; and, if so, whether such policies would properly balance the need for public safety with the right of individual autonomy.

It is perhaps the highest goal of the law to protect the right of individuals to autonomy and self-determination. Traditionally three groups have been excluded from this protection—children, the mentally ill and retarded, and those harboring infectious disease. It is only recently that lawyers have given any careful thought to the first two of these groups. The third—carriers of infectious disease—has remained, for the most part, a throw away line in the legal literature.

The courts have shown considerable deference to the exercise of the state's police power to promote the public health. The Supreme Court in *Jacobson v. Massachusetts*[59] held that Massachusetts law that enabled local health authorities to require vaccination was constitutional. As between individual autonomy and the common good of the people, the latter constituted an overriding interest. The court did establish limits which required that the state refrain from acting in "an arbitrary, unreasonable manner," or "going so far beyond what was reasonably required for the safety of the public." The public health power, then, must have a "real or substantial relation" to public health objectives and not be so sweeping as to interfere needlessly with personal liberty or autonomy.

This concept of medical necessity in the exercise of public health powers remains to the present.[60] Yet courts have very rarely imposed any substantive boundaries on the measures which can be taken. The courts have upheld public health powers ranging from immunization,[59,60] compulsory examination and treatment,[61] to quarantine.[62] Quarantine amounts to compulsory deprivation of liberty and should attract the greatest judicial protection. Yet courts have repeatedly upheld quarantine during periods of epidemics—veneral disease, typhoid, tuberculosis, smallpox, scarlet fever, leprosy, cholera, and bubonic plague.

Judicial scrutiny of quarantine law has not reflected even the minimal substantive limitations against irrational or overreaching powers as set by the Supreme Court. In *Kirk v. Wyman*,[63] the court upheld a local health authority's decision to quarantine an elderly woman with aesthetic leprosy, a disease which was acknowledged to pose "hardly any danger of contagion." There was no evidence that she had transmitted the disease to anyone during her many years in the community. Miss Kirk's disease was incurable and her quarantine persisted for life. Mary Mallon, the legendary typhoid fever carrier of the early 20th century, was quarantined on an island for 23 years until her death.[64]

So too have the courts refused to interfere even when the actions of public health officials were not clearly focused on preventable harm. Decisions by public health officials to detain and treat those suspected of having venereal disease were regularly upheld, even in the absence of a prior judicial determination that the person had the infection and was likely to engage in behavior likely to transmit it to others. Alleged prostitutes "reasonably suspected" of having venereal disease[65] were considered "natural subjects and carriers," making it "logical and natural that suspicion be cast upon them and necessity dictate a physical examination of their persons."[66]

The courts, then, have deferred to public health measures even where they resulted in indefinite confinement and despite inconclusive evidence of a tangible public health benefit. But it would be a mistake to assume future judicial complacency in reviewing compulsory powers against AIDS patients. Almost all of the relevant cases were decided during a period which preceded the evolution in construction of the Fourteenth Amendment.

Previously, so long as a classification was not based upon race,[67] national origin,[68] or alienage,[69] it was reviewed under a standard of minimum rationality—provided the legislature had not acted arbitrarily or without any reasonable basis, the public health measure would be upheld. Equal protection analysis now incorporates heightened standards of review beyond minimum rationality. Where the statute impinges on a fundamental right, such as liberty,[70] the state must demonstrate a compelling interest and show that the means used are the least restrictive necessary to accomplish that statutory objective.[71] Once the highest standard of review is triggered it has virtually become a signal that the courts will not uphold the statute. A middle tier of scrutiny[72] is involved where important, but less than fundamental rights are infringed. Here the courts require "exceedingly persuasive justification," and means which are substantially related to the state objective.[73]

While it is well-settled that liberty and travel interests trigger the strictest Fourteenth Amendment scrutiny,[70] there are two possible avenues of constitutional analyses relevant to AIDS which are less clear. First, there have been persuasive arguments that homosexuality should be a quasi-suspect classification as it is inborn, inalienable, and stigmatic; gays are an insular minority with a long history of discrimination.[74] The courts have yet to accept or reject this argument but the characteristics of the class do warrant special attention. Second, the courts have held that constitutionally protected privacy interests may be involved where there is potential "disclosure of personal matters."[75] Privacy is not directly guaranteed in the Constitution but is built upon a penumbra of constitutional guarantees; it is difficult to predict, therefore, where the courts might find constitutionally protected privacy interests.[76]

This evolution of equal protection analysis since the early public health cases suggests that those cases are unreliable precedent for contemporary analysis of AIDS legislation. More representative of current constitutional analysis is to be found in *New York State Association for Retarded Children v. Carey*[77] concerning the highly analogous disease, hepatitis B, which is transmitted in much the same way as the AIDS-related virus. The court determined that mentally retarded children who were carriers of serum hepatitis could not be excluded from attending regular public school classes. Hepatitis B is transmitted by blood and, although the virus is found on saliva, it is an extremely inefficient mode of transmission. The court found that "the Board was unable to demonstrate that the health hazard . . . was anything more than a remote possibility." This remote possibility did not justify the action taken considering "the detrimental effects of isolating the carrier children." The court was sensitive to the fact that segregation of mentally retarded children would "reinforce the stigma to which these children have already been subjected."[78]

Even where courts accede to the power of state legislatures to protect the public health they may require procedural due process safeguards prior to or immediately after the use of control measures. Strict due process standards for quarantines are necessary because fundamental freedoms are at stake; there is a distinct risk of erroneous fact finding; and there is no state interest in confining nondangerous individuals.

The West Virginia supreme court has held that the same procedural safeguards required in civil commitment to mental hospitals are applicable in cases of involuntary confinement of infectious patients. These procedures include written notice, counsel, presenting evidence and cross examination, a clear and convincing standard of proof, and a verbatim transcript for appeal.[79]

There follows an analysis of how today's courts would be likely to review reporting and registration requirements and quarantines of AIDS patients or carriers.

Reporting and Registers. The constitutional dimensions of reporting and maintaining registers of infectious disease depends upon the procedures and objectives of measures. They need not heavily impinge upon the interests of individuals as long as public health officials are not required to provide names and intimate information such as sexual contacts on the registry. Thus, under current national requirements for reporting "full blown" AIDS, where names are kept purely for epidemiologic purposes and where confidentiality is assured, the privacy interest of any individual on the register is minimal. It is quite clear that the courts would support narrowly conceived public measures such as this. It would be otherwise if personal information were to be disclosed outside the Public Health Service, or if information were collected in order to implement other control measures; in the latter case any individual interest affected would depend upon the measure to be implemented.

This introduction has already drawn attention to the justification for reporting the disease state and not the carrier status, *i.e.*, the precision, objectivity, and reliability of the disease state can be far better assured than the carrier state. Accordingly, statistical objectives can be achieved by the more limited disease reporting requirement.

Jurisdictions such as Colorado require reporting of the carrier status. Carriers can transmit the virus at least as effectively as those with the disease; patients with full blown AIDS are less likely to engage fully in normal life, including sexual activities, than are asymptomatic carriers. However, reporting all carriers requires the collection of a mass of highly personal information with all the risk of intentional or negligent disclosure and all the consequent disincentives to people seeking testing and counseling. Moreover, nothing can be done with this information which would further any public health objective. If there were a vaccination or treatment to arrest the disease process this information would be invaluable. But given the current state of the science, collection of this information would be based upon irrational prejudice and might well be struck down by a court, particularly if there were a real risk of information on the register being disclosed.

Judicial analysis, then, would balance the magnitude of the public health benefits to be achieved against the intrusion on the personal interests of the AIDS patient or carrier. Where sensitive information is collected including names, addresses, and personal contacts, and where the confidentiality safeguards are inadequate, privacy interests might be compromised. In such circumstances the courts would not countenance a reporting measure which was more sweeping or intrusive than necessary and where the legislature had no compelling public health purpose.

Quarantine.   The constitutional objections to a general quarantine are potentially insurmountable. Quarantines directly infringe upon a person's liberty. It is a uniquely serious form of deprivation as it can be utilized against a competent person; it is based upon what a person might do in the future rather than what he or she has done; there is no clear limitation of time; and it is not subject to the same vigorous due process procedures as in crime. Given the impact on liberty and travel, quarantine is likely to trigger the highest equal protection scrutiny. This means that the legislation must be narrowly tailored to achieve a compelling public interest, and must be the least restrictive and least intrusive measure necessary to achieve that objective.

General quarantines which applied to all those with the disease or those who tested positive for HTLV-III antibodies would not be constitutionally acceptable. Deprivation of liberty based upon a disease or viral status would be substantially overbroad: not all those who test positive harbor the live virus; even if a reliable test for the live virus could be found, it would be impossible to predict their future behavior leading to transmission of the virus. Given the inability to determine who would, and would not, communicate the disease, deprivation of liberty of entire population groups could not be accepted.

There are numerous public policy reasons against a general quarantine that flow from the unique combination of scientific findings which set AIDS apart from other quarantinable infectious diseases: the sheer magnitude of the number of people capable of communicating the virus, which at present approaches one million; there is no incubation period so that the period of infectiousness, and consequently of the quarantine itself, would be without limit of time; there is no prevention or treatment so that those quarantined would have no way to restore themselves back to a normal condition in order to rejoin the community; and, the virus is not spread through casual contact, making segregation from society unnecessary and invidious. The state of the science of AIDS, then, should completely rule out a general quarantine as a viable policy option at present.

More limited quarantines suffer from many of the same public policy objections. Nevertheless they might not attract judicial censure. Allowable quarantine statutes would not focus on a person's *status* as having an infection or disease, but upon his or her *behavior* leading to transmission. A quarantine statute could require public health officials to determine that the person harboring the AIDS-related virus is unwilling or unable to refrain from engaging in activity likely to spread the disease. The impact on a person's liberty interest would result in the strictest judicial scrutiny. Still, the state could point to a narrowly tailored means of preventing spread of the disease in each individual case. The courts conceivably could find this sufficiently compelling to support the quarantine.

If a public health official has good reason to believe that a person is recalcitrant and will continue to engage sexual partners, it is difficult to see the courts leaving the state with no stick to ensure compliant behavior.

Even if the courts were to uphold limited quarantines, there are distinct public policy difficulties which make them weak candidates for implementation. First, any kind of compulsory measure which is as drastic as deprivation of liberty may discourage individuals from seeking testing or treatment, or speaking honestly to counselors concerning their future behavioral intentions. Second, it would be exceedingly difficult to frame objective criteria to determine future dangerousness. It is difficult, almost impossible, to predict who will and will not engage in dangerous behavior. A declared intention to engage in such behavior cannot be distinguished from others who foreswear unsafe activity. Third, those who come to the attention of public health officials are likely to be the poorest, least articulate of those harboring the virus; the vast majority of instances of transmission will surely go unnoticed. This makes a limited quarantine a kind of a lottery affecting primarily the most vulnerable and having the most negligible impact on the epidemiology of the disease. Finally, introducing a quarantine based upon preventing intimate behavior has unimaginable monitoring and enforcement difficulties. It could be viewed as a license for public health and law enforcement officials to intrude into the most private parts of people's lives.

Less restrictive alternatives might well be preferable as public health options if *any* control measures were thought necessary over and above voluntary persuasion. These less restrictive alternatives might include supervision orders with fines for noncompliance or requirements of daily attendance at courses or at health care or law enforcement facilities, or guardianship of incompetent patients.

Meritorious of some consideration could be a public health statute for knowingly engaging in behavior likely to transmit the virus. This is preferable to quarantine because it clearly places the individual on notice of the behavior which is proscribed; it is based upon what a person has done, not what he might do in the future; it has strict due process safeguards; and, it has a finite period of incarceration. While society may well wish to establish some formal sanction for dangerous behavior it seeks to discourage, many of the same disadvantages of a limited quarantine apply in this case. The major issues involve the intrusion of enforcement, the difficulties of proof, and the disincentive to seeking voluntary testing, counseling, and care.

Conclusion

This introduction is only a preliminary examination of a full range of public policy questions posed by the alarming spread of AIDS; a more complete study is in process. The state of the science at present is evolving but public policymakers must not make leaps of logic to presume future scenarios which cannot currently be predicted. The current state of the science is that the AIDS-related virus is exceedingly difficult to transmit—realistically, only by direct exchange of body fluids. Policy must strictly adhere to the facts and not allow panic or irrational prejudice to influence policy decisions. This is especially so where wrong decisions impose unconscionable restrictions on the rights of individuals and groups historically discriminated against.

References

1. Message from Secretary Heckler and Letter from Commissioner Young. 1985. *FDA Drug Bulletin* 15:26.
2. Centers for Disease Control. 1981. Pneumocystis Pneumonia—Los Angeles. *Morbidity and Mortality Weekly Report* 30:250-2.
3. Centers for Disease Control. 1981. Kaposi's sarcoma and pneumocystis pneumonia among homosexual men. *Morbidity and Mortality Weekly Report* 25:305-8.
4. Centers for Disease Control. 1982. Update on acquired immune deficiency syndrome (AIDS)—United States. *Morbidity and Mortality Weekly Report* 31:507-14.
5. World Health Organization. 1985. Acquired Immune Deficiency Syndrome: Meeting of the WHO laboratory centres on AIDS. *Weekly Epidemiological Record* 43:333-4; 35:270-1.
6. Diagnoses are considered to fit the case definition only if based on sufficiently reliable methods (generally histology or culture).
7. The CDC list of "moderately indicative" diseases is broken down into five etiologic categories and includes pneumocystis carinii pneumonia, toxoplasmosis, candidiasis, herpes simplex virus, and Kaposi's sarcoma.
8. The CDC definition was consolidated in Selik, R.M., Haverkos, and J.W. Curran. 1984. Acquired immune deficiency syndrome (AIDS) trends in the United States 1978–1982. *American Journal of Medicine* 76:493-500. Several amendments (e.g., Jaffee, H.W., D.J. Bregman, and R.M. Selik. 1983. Acquired immune deficiency syndrome in the United States: the first 1,000 cases. *Journal of Infectious Diseases* 148:339-45) and deletions (Jaffee, H.W., and R.M. Selik. Acquired immune deficiency syndrome: a disseminated aspergillosis predictive of underlying cellular immune deficiency? *Journal of Infectious Diseases* 149:829) had previously been made.
9. Centers for Disease Control. 1985. Revision of the case definition of acquired immune deficiency syndrome for national reporting—United States. *Morbidity and Mortality Weekly Report* 34:373-5. The CDC definition does not apply to children under age 10 but a pro-

visional definition has been developed. Centers for Disease Control. 1984. Update: acquired immune deficiency syndrome (AIDS)—United States. *Morbidity and Mortality Weekly Report* 32:688–91.

10. Weiss, S.H., J.J. Goedert, M.G. Sarngadharan, et al. 1985. Screening test for HTLV-III (AIDS agent) antibodies: specificity, sensitivity, and applications. *Journal of the American Medical Association* 253: 221–5.

11. Goedert, J., and W. Blattner. 1985. The epidemiology of the acquired immune deficiency syndrome. In: *AIDS*, ed. V.T. DeVita, S. Hellman, and S.A. Rosenberg. Philadelphia: J.B. Lippincott.

12. Shaw, G.M., M.E. Harper, B.H. Hahn, et al. 1985. HTLV-III infection in brains of children and adults with AIDS encephalopathy. *Science* 227:177–82.

13. Ammann, A.J. 1985. The acquired immune deficiency syndrome in infants and children. *Annals of Internal Medicine* 103:734–7.

14. Curran, J.W., W. Meade Morgan, A.M. Hardy, et al. 1985. The epidemiology of AIDS: current status and future prospects. *Science* 229: 1352–7.

15. Sandberg, S., and H. Sherman. 1985. Mathematical Model of the AIDS Epidemic. Unpublished study sponsored by the Massachusetts Department of Public Health.

16. Gallo, R.C., S.Z. Salahuddin, M. Popouic, et al. 1984. Frequent detection and isolation of cytopathic retroviruses (HTLV-III) from patients with AIDS and at risk for AIDS. *Science* 224:500–3.

17. Popovic, M., M.G. Sarngadharan, E. Read, and R.C. Gallo. 1984. Detection, isolation, and continuous production of cytopathic retroviruses (HTLV-III) from patients with AIDS and pre-AIDS. *Science* 224:497–500.

18. Barre-Sinoussi, F., J.C. Chermann, and F. Rey, et al. 1983. Isolation of a T-lymphotropic retrovirus from a patient at risk for acquired immune deficiency syndrome (AIDS). *Science* 220:868–71.

19. Barre-Sinoussi, F., U. Mathur-Wagh, F. Rey, et al. 1985. Isolation of lymphadenopathy associated virus (LAV) and detection of LAV antibodies from U.S. patients with AIDS. *Journal of the American Medical Association* 253:1737–9.

20. Levy, J.A., A.D. Hoffman, S.M. Kramer, et al. 1983. Isolation of lymphocytopathic retroviruses from San Francisco patients with AIDS. *Science* 255:840–2.

21. Special report: the AIDS epidemic. 1985. *New England Journal of Medicine* 312:521–5.

22. Sarngadharan, M.G., M. Popouic, L. Bruch, et al. 1984. Antibodies reactive with human T-lymphotropic retrovirus (HTLV-III) in the serum of patients with AIDS. *Science* 224:506–8.

23. Petricciani, J.C. 1985. Licensed tests for antibody to human T-lymphotropic virus type III: sensitivity and specificity. *Annals of Internal Medicine* 103:726–9.

24. Schorrs, B., A. Berkowitz, P.D. Cumming, et al. 1985. Prevalence of HTLV-III antibody in American blood donors. *New England Journal of Medicine* 313:384–5.

25. See generally Levine, C., and R. Bayer. 1985. Screening blood: public health and medical uncertainty. In a special supplement entitled AIDS: the emerging ethical dilemmas. *Hastings Center Report* 15(4):8–11. Marwick, C. 1985. Use of AIDS antibody test may provide more answers. *Journal of the American Medical Association* 253:1694–9; Osterholm, M.T., R.J. Bowman, M.W. Chopek, et al. 1985. Screening donated blood from plasma for HTLV-III anti-

body: Facing one more crisis. *New England Journal of Medicine* 312: 1185–9.

26. Evatt, B.L., E.D. Gomperts, J.S. Mc-Dougal, and R.B. Ramsey. 1985. Incidental appearance of LAV/HTLV-III antibodies in hemophiliacs and the onset of the AIDS epidemic. *New England Journal of Medicine* 312:483–6.

27. Goedert, J.J., M.E. Eyster, M.G. Sarngadharan, et al. 1985. Antibodies reactive with human T-cell leukemia viruses in the serum of hemophiliacs receiving factor VIII concentrate. *Blood* 65:492–5.

28. Melbye, M., K.S. Froebel, R. Madhok, et al. 1984. HTLV-III seropositivity in European hemophiliacs exposed to factor VIII concentrate imported from the USA. *Lancet* 2:1444–6.

29. Eyster, M.E., J.J. Goedert, M.G. Sarngadharan, et al. 1985. Development and early natural history of HTLV-III antibodies in persons with hemophilia. *Journal of the American Medical Association* 253:2219–23.

30. Centers for Disease Control. 1984. Antibodies to a retrovirus etiologically associated with acquired immune deficiency syndrome (AIDS) in populations with increased incidences of the syndrome. *Morbidity and Mortality Weekly Report* 33:377–9.

31. Centers for Disease Control. 1985. Results of human T-lymphotropic virus type III test kits reported from blood collection centers—U.S., April 22–May 19, 1985. *Morbidity and Mortality Weekly Report* 34:375–76. See similar studies reported in: Progress on AIDS. 1985. *FDA Drug Bulletin* 15:27–32.

32. In one CDC/American Red Cross study, strongly and repeatedly reactive blood units correlated highly with both positive Western blot tests (94%) and positive culture for HTLV-III (50%); 89% were found to be in identifiable risk groups. Still, of the approximately 3 in 1,200 blood donors found to be repeatedly reactive, only about 1 in 1,200 will likely be infected with HTLV-III. Allen J.R., et al. 1985. HTLV-III antibody screening in a blood bank: laboratory and chemical correlations. Proceedings of Workshop on Experience with HTLV-III Antibody Testing, sponsored by FDA, NIH, and CDC, July 31.

33. Young, F.E. 1985. Commissioner of Food and Drugs, "Dear Doctor" Letter. February 19.

34. Ho, D.D., R.T. Schooley, T.A. Rota, et al. 1984. HTLV-III in the semen and blood of a healthy homosexual man. *Science* 226:451–3.

35. Zagury, D., J. Bernard, J. Leibowitch, et al. 1984. HTLV-III in cells cultured from semen of two patients with AIDS. *Science* 226:449–51.

36. Groopman, J.E., S.Z. Salahuddin, M.G. Sarngadharan, et al. 1984. HTLV-III in saliva of people with AIDS-related complex and healthy homosexual men at risk for AIDS. *Science* 226:447–8.

37. Fajikawa, L.S., S.Z. Salahuddin, A.G. Palestine, et al. 1985. Isolation of human T-cell leukemia/lymphototropic virus type III (HTLV-III) from the tears of a patient with acquired immune deficiency syndrome (AIDS). *Lancet* 2:529.

38. Redfield, R.R., P.D. Markham, S.Z. Salahuddin, et al. 1985. Heterosexually acquired HTLV-III/LAV disease (AIDS-related complex and AIDS): Epidemiologic evidence for female to male transmission. *Journal of the American Medical Association* 254:2094–6.

39. Centers for Disease Control. 1985. Heterosexual transmission of human T-lymphotropic virus type III/lymphadenopathy associated virus. *Morbidity and Mortality Weekly Report* 34:561–3.

40. Piet, P., T.C. Quinn, H. Taelman, et al. 1984. Acquired immune deficiency syndrome in a heterosexual population in Zaire. *Lancet* 2:65–9.

41. Clumeck, N., P. van de Perre, M. Cargel, et al. 1985. Heterosexual promiscuity among African patients with AIDS. *New England Journal of Medicine* 313:182.

42. Redfield, R.R., P.D. Markham, S.Z. Salahuddin, et al. 1985. Frequent transmission of HTLV-III among spouses of patients with AIDS-related complex and AIDS. *Journal of the American Medical Association* 253:1571–3.

43. Blumberg, B.S., and R.C. Fox. 1985. The Daedalus effect: Changes in ethical questions relating to hepatitis B. *Annals of Internal Medicine* 102:390–4.

44. Centers for Disease Control. 1985. Self-reported behavior change among gay and bisexual men—San Francisco. *Morbidity and Mortality Weekly Report* 34(40):613–5; Schecter, M.T., E. Jeffries, P. Constance, et al. 1984. Changes in sexual behavior and fear of AIDS. *Lancet* 1:1293; Centers for Disease Control. 1984. Declining rates of rectal and pharyngeal gonorrhea among males—NYC. *Morbidity and Mortality Weekly Report* 33:295–7.

45. Brandt, A.M. 1985. No magic bullet: A social history of veneral disease in the United States since 1880. New York: Oxford University Press.

46. Curran, W.J. 1975. Venereal disease detention and treatment: Prostitution and civil rights. *American Journal of Public Health* 65(2): 180–1.

47. See government recommendations for behavior change on voluntary basis. Centers for Disease Control. 1983. Prevention of acquired immune deficiency syndrome (AIDS): Report of interagency recommendations. *Morbidity and Mortality Weekly Report* 32:101–3.

48. *Tarasoff v. The Regents of the University of California*, 118 Cal. Rptr. 192, 529 P.2d 553 (1975).

49. Centers for Disease Control. 1985. Provisional Public Health Service inter-agency recommendations for screening donated blood and plasma for antibody to virus causing acquired immune deficiency syndrome. *Morbidity and Mortality Weekly Report* 34(1):1–5.

50. See *Alberts v. Devine*, 395 Mass. 59 (1985).

51. 42 CFR Part 2, 42 U.S.C. §242K, §242M, 49 *Federal Register* 48998 (December 17, 1984).

52. Consideration would have to be given as to whether federal regulations could reach the activities of a private agency not reliant on federal funding. Cf. *Irwin Memorial Blood Bank v. American National Red Cross*, 640 F.2d 1051 (1981).

53. See *Cronin v. Strayer*, 392 Mass. 525 (1984).

54. *South Florida Blood Service, Inc. v. Rasmussen*, 467 So.2d 798 (Fla. 3d DCA 1985); cert. granted (Fla.S.Ct. Case No. 67,081).

55. Weiss, S.H., W.C. Saxinger, D. Rechtman, et al. 1985. HTLV-III infection among health care workers: Association with needle-stick injuries. *Journal of the American Medical Association* 254:2089–93.

56. Centers for Disease Control. 1985. Update: prospective evaluation of health care workers exposed via the parenteral or mucous-membrane

route to body fluids from patients with acquired immune deficiency syndrome—United States. *Morbidity and Mortality Weekly Report* 34:101-3.

57. Centers for Disease Control. 1982. Acquired immune deficiency syndrome (AIDS): Precautions for clinical and laboratory staff. *Morbidity and Mortality Weekly Report* 31:577-80.

58. Centers for Disease Control. 1983. Acquired immune deficiency syndrome (AIDS): Precautions for health-care workers and allied proposals. *Morbidity and Mortality Weekly Report* 32:450-1.

59. *Jacobson v. Massachusetts*, 197 U.S. 11 (1905).

60. See *Application of the President and Directors of Georgetown College, Inc.*, 331 F.2d 1000, at 1008 ("It has been firmly established . . . that adults, sick or well, can be required to submit to compulsory treatment or prophylaxis"). *Prince v. Massachusetts*, 321 U.S. 158 at 166-67 (1944) ("The right to practice religion freely does not include liberty to expose the community or the child to communicable disease.").

61. *Welch v. Shepherd*, 165 Kan. 394, 196 P.2d 235 (1948); *Ex parte King*, 128 Cal. App. 27, 16 P.2d 694 (1932); *Ex parte Company*, 106 Ohio St. 50, 139 N.E. 204 (1922); *State v. Snow*, 324 S.W.2d 532 (1959).

62. *People v. Robertson*, 302 Ill. 422, 134 N.E. 815 (1922); *Compagnie Francaise de Navigation a Vapeur*, 186 U.S. 380 (1902). *State v. Rackowski*, 86A 606 (1913).

63. 83 S.C. 372, 65 S.E. 387 (1909).

64. Soper. 1939. The curious case of Typhoid Mary. *Bulletin of the New York Academy of Medicine* 15:698.

65. *Ex parte Company*, 139 N.E. at 205.

66. *People v. Strautz*, 386 Ill. 360, 54 N.E.2d 441, 444 (1944).

67. *Korematsu v. United States*, 323 U.S. 214 (1944).

68. See *Oyama v. California*, 332 U.S. 633 (1948).

69. See *Graham v. Richardson*, 403 U.S. 369 (1971).

70. See *Shapiro v. Thompson*, 394 U.S. 618 (1969).

71. *Dunn v. Blumstein*, 405 U.S. 330 at 342.

72. E.g., *Reed v. Reed*, 404 U.S. 71 (1971) (gender). See Note, Refining the methods of middle-tier scrutiny: A new proposal for equal protection, 61 *Texas Law Review* 1501 (1983).

73. *Mississippi University for Women v. Hogan*, 458 U.S. 718, 724 (1981).

74. Note, The Constitutional Status of Sexual Orientation: Homosexuality as a Suspect Classification, 98 *Harvard Law Review* 1285 (1985); Note, An Argument for the Application of Equal Protection Heightened Scrutiny to Classifications Based on Homosexuality, 57 *Southern California Law Review* 797 (1984).

75. *Whalen v. Roe*, 97 S.Ct. 869 (1977).

76. See *State v. Saunders*, 381 A.2d 333 (1977) (state's interests in preventing venereal disease found insufficient to justify fornication statute's impingement on privacy).

77. 612 F.2d 644 (2d Cir. 1979).

78. 612 F.2d at 650-51.

79. *Greene v. Edwards*, 263 S.E.2d 661 (1980).

PART II
Public Health Response to the AIDS Crisis

Addressing Public Health Concerns of the City of San Francisco

Mervyn Silverman, M.D.
Consultant and former Director of the San Francisco
Department of Public Health

The history of medicine is replete with tragic epidemics affecting the lives of literally hundreds of thousands of individuals. Over the last hundred years, however, no disease has been so complex, or has so challenged the medical community, as the acquired immune deficiency syndrome, or AIDS. At the same time, seemingly insolvable moral problems, legal problems, and complex social ramifications are raised. These various issues represent significant areas of concern that have consumed a great deal of my time over the last three years.

As we all know, AIDS is a worldwide health crisis affecting people inhabiting almost every continent. The first cases in the United States were reported in 1981, and as of 2 September 1985, 12,932 cases have been diagnosed. Over 50% of these individuals have died.[1] It has been estimated that the number of diagnosed cases will double in such a way that the cases diagnosed in 1986 alone will equal all of the cases that have been diagnosed since 1978.

As to the origin of this disease, we must look to equatorial Africa where, according to present knowledge, the incidence of AIDS predates all other areas of the world. The association between AIDS and central Africa was first noted after Belgian and French physicians observed that an AIDS-like illness existed in Africans from Zaire and Rwanda who were living in Europe at that time. These cases were first observed in the late 1970s. Is this a new disease, or is it possible that the infectious agent causing AIDS has been endemic in Africa, and has gone unrecognized for years until it recently became disseminated into other populations? It is unlikely that these questions will ever be totally answered, but there is evidence suggesting that the present *high* incidence of AIDS in Zaire, Rwanda, and Kenya is a relatively recent phenomenon. Recent studies have shown that of those patients studied in Zaire, 12% tested positive to the HTLV-III antibody test; in Kenya approximately 20% tested positive.[2]

Retrospective analyses of case records of patients seem to indicate that AIDS has been present in Zaire since at least 1972, suggesting a spread from Zaire to the United States and Haiti. Two important differences exist, however, between AIDS in Africa and AIDS in Europe and the United States. First, in Africa the numbers of men and women with this disease are roughly equal; the ratio of men to women in the United States is approximately 14 to 1. Second, in Africa, there is an apparent lack of the risk factors that have been identified in the United States, such as homosexuality, IV drug abuse, or a history of blood-product transfusions. Frequent injection with possibly unsterilized needles and syringes, a practice of scarification, and poor hygiene during medical procedures may play an important role in the transmission of the AIDS agent in these countries. As discussed in the Atlanta conference on AIDS, one study suggests that a special variety of monkey that inhabits the areas of Africa under consideration has an infection very much like AIDS.[3] The monkeys are cross-reactive to the HTLV-III antibody. They appear to tolerate it quite well, however. It is possible that the virus was transmitted initially from animal to human through a bite of some sort.

If we presume that the disease is indigenous to these monkeys in Africa, then why are patients dying from the disease now, as opposed to a millennium ago? We cannot be certain as to what natural or unnatural event is responsible for the development of this invasive, parasitic infection. Some unusual event thrust the human vector into contact with the virus in a manner not encountered before. There are several ecologic precedents for this theory. For example, supposedly in the 1930s, a woman visiting Cairo, Egypt, became enamored with an Egyptian plant, the water hyacinth. This was prior to the restrictions imposed by the United States on bringing plants back to the United States. She brought the water hyacinths back to Florida, planted them in her back yard where a stream was going through her property. It is now estimated that almost all the waterways of Florida are clogged with water hyacinths. Water hyacinths have been described in ancient Egypt thousands of years ago; waterways in Florida have been around for thousands of years. Something took place which brought them together resulting in a very serious ecologic problem.

What we do not know about AIDS at this time is what happened to cause the parasitic virus to invade the human host. In Africa, since colonial times, there have been extensive social dislocations of the populations that reside there. New roads have been opening to outsiders into some very rural areas. As the ecomomy of Africa changes, as more urbanization and crowding in the cities occurs, it may be that diseases such as AIDS or infectious organisms such as HTLV-III or something else endemic in the rural areas of Africa could have gone unnoticed. If someone dies of pneumonia or cancer in a rural area, the facilities to perform sophisticated laboratory analysis to determine if a T-cell deficiency is present in a patient in these areas may be lacking. Any of these possibilities for the recent onset of AIDS as a deadly disease are conceivable; we will have to devote more research time and resources to elucidate the cause.

AIDS was probably introduced into Haiti from the United States by vacationing American homosexuals, as the island was recognized as a well-known and fashionable resort throughout the late 1970s. It is felt that if AIDS had been prevalent in Haiti for any significant period of time, one would have expected cases to occur in the neighboring Dominican Republic, which has not been the case.

The clinical scenario of a patient debilitated with AIDS is quite similar around the world. When the number of patients with the disease began to increase, however, it became evident that the diagnosis of AIDS itself represented only the extreme end of the clinical spectrum of the disease. AIDS is defined by the Centers for Disease Control (CDC) an an opportunistic infection or malignancy, predictive of cellular immune deficiency in a person under age 60 who has no underlying immunosuppressive condition.[4]

At this time the disease is considered to be universally fatal. The typical AIDS patient is a homosexual or bisexual male between the ages of 25 and 45, who lives in a large city and has been sexually active. This represents about 73% of the cases nationwide.[5] The next largest subset of cases is found in IV drug abusers (17%). Patients who have received blood transfusions (2%), hemophiliacs (1%), and the sexual partners of persons from the AIDS risk groups (1%) are a small percentage of those patients affected. The other few percentage points are in those patients that have to be classified as unknown, because the people have either died with their risk factors undetermined, or it is unclear why they contracted the disease. These people represent a very small percentage of the patients in this category.

The Haitians no longer are considered to be at higher risk than other members of the population. These patients in the Haitian community with AIDS had high risk factors because of their sexual activity or IV drug abuse, no different really than those in other communities or countries where people with AIDS are in the high risk group.

One thing that is interesting, as the history of this disease over the last three or so years is reviewed, is that the percentages of the people in these various groups have remained relatively constant, an apparent fact that is most important. The disease has not been expanding dramatically outside the expected high risk groups. We have seen, however, more than 70 cases of infants with AIDS born to high risk mothers and infants of mothers who have had contact with persons in the high risk groups.

We presently believe that the cause of AIDS is a variant of a known human cancer retrovirus. This variant is called HTLV-III, or human T-cell lymphotrophic virus. HTLV-III and LAV, lymphadenopathy-associated virus, which was isolated in France, appear to be the same virus. They are both retroviruses, and are so named for their ability to convert RNA, ribonucleic acid, into DNA, deoxyribonucleic acid, the hereditary chemicals which make up the genes of human and animal cells. In so doing, these viruses use the genetic machinery of the cells they infect to make the protein they need for survival. In the process, there is a profound impairment of the cell-mediated immunity, which is that part of the body's immune system responsible for host defense against viruses, intracellular organisms, and tumor antigens. Once infected, the incubation or latency period can range from a matter of months to five or more years. One study discussed in Atlanta using mathematical modeling indicates that the latency or incubation period could continue for as long as 14 years.[6]

In general, AIDS is suspected when a physician is confronted with a high risk patient having no underlying cause of immune deficiency, who presents signs and symptoms of an opportunistic infection or malignancy such as pneumocystis carinii pneumonia or Kaposi's sarcoma. By 1982, chronic generalized lymph node enlargement and other nonspecific symptoms were known to be much more common than AIDS among the high risk groups. In other words, since the discovery of the AIDS virus, it has become obvious that the clinical manifestations of classical AIDS represents only the tip of an iceberg. Based on studies done in San Francisco, it is estimated that the number of persons who have been infected in the United States is between 300,000 and 1,000,000.[1] Of the 10,000 or more cases of AIDS which will be diagnosed during the next year, this tip of the iceberg will represent only 1% or 2% of those currently infected. It is thus reasonable to assume that the number of persons infected with the virus in many areas of the United States probably exceeds by a hundredfold those who have been reported with AIDS. Current studies indicate that among homosexual men who have been infected with the HTLV-III or LAV virus, between 5% and 20% will develop AIDS within the first two to five years of infection, and more than half of those infected will remain without symptoms for a prolonged period. One study identified 20 homosexual men who had been infected with the virus for two to six years and yet had remained asymptomatic; the authors were able to isolate the virus from a single specimen of blood in 60% of these cases. The viral infection can thus persist for many years, and perhaps last a lifetime. We must therefore consider a positive antibody test as evidence of current infection until specific tests are available for the antigen or the virus. We must also assume that those with positive tests can transmit the infection to others through sexual contact or by way of blood contamination. Because of a low prevalence of infection in the general population, and fewer sexual partners, it is likely that the heterosexual spread of infection will not be as rapid as the spread among homosexuals, IV drug abusers, or persons with hemophilia.

An increase in heterosexual transmission in the United States is inevitable. Those who use IV drugs, engage in prostitution, or who have very large numbers of heterosexual partners will be at the highest risk of acquiring and transmitting the disease. One thing that I think we all know and should really emphasize is that it is not a disease that is spread by casual contact. Normal human daily contact is not going to spread the disease.

The first cases of AIDS in San Francisco were diagnosed in 1981. In July, 1981, the City of San Francisco established a reporting and case registry system for AIDS. The cases that have been reported have been investigated and the patients interviewed, where possible, with liaison being established between the Department of Public Health, various hospitals, private physicians' offices, and the Centers for Disease Control. In October, 1982, the City's Department of Public Health established the multidisciplinary AIDS clinic at San Francisco

General Hospital that allowed for AIDS screening, diagnosis, treatment, follow-up, education, and counseling. As the number of cases increased, other screening clinics were established throughout the city. The first inpatient ward for AIDS cases was opened in 1983, also at San Francisco General Hospital. At the outset of the opening of that unit, I became quite concerned that we might be isolating the patient from family, friends, and other support systems, setting up a leper colony type of situation. I was relieved to discover that I was quite wrong; we had more professionals and other staff applying to work on the unit than there were available positions. The AIDS unit has proved to be an incredible success from both the medical aspect and, especially, from the social and psychological aspects of the disease. Comments from patients such as "I feel secure," "I feel safe," are commonplace. Each patient is assigned to a social services counselor who helps them address their needs. Other counselors, both professional and lay practitioners, work with patients, worried well persons, loved ones, and others. The unit is in the process of being expanded to a 30-bed unit; the concept is being replicated in several other areas around the United States.

Education and training was, at the outset, considered to be a very important aspect of the program. In cooperation with gay organizations, more than 500,000 pieces of literature, to both the gay and general population, were distributed during the first year of the program. The consciousness of these communities has been enhanced by these and other educational efforts. One of the first educational posters that we developed was considered quite radical in 1982, so radical, in fact, that at a gay meeting in Denver, it was booed and hissed. The notice basically said, "Limit the number of sexual partners, reduce the use of drugs, and don't share body fluids." Today, this notice would not generate the same type of response from the gay community. The social and psychologic dynamics of the disease are radically changing over time. More than 500 training sessions, educational programs, and forums have been held, and a hotline has been established over which thousands of calls have been received. Signs have been posted in buses and bars; public service announcements have been placed on television and radio. These services were being provided at a time when the hysteria in the general community was rising at an unprecedented rate and to an unprecedented level. It seems as though the more we attempted to calm the fear, the greater the problems of misunderstanding and hysteria became. At that time, the cause of the disease and the mode of transmission was unknown, there was (and is) no cure, there was (and is) no vaccine, and it was universally fatal. Perhaps the reason the fears have abated somewhat is due to the efforts of many groups whose express purpose was to educate people about the disease, and to calm the possibly not irrational but perhaps unnecessary fears.

Over the last five or six years, we have worked with a lesbian–gay coordinating committee to address the health needs of the gay community. This committee gathered and distributed resource materials to the professional community. An

AIDS Task Force and an AIDS Medical Advisory Group were established. Representatives from blood banks, the University of California at San Francisco Medical Center, epidemiologists, psychologists, and community members, both gay and straight, participated.

Once the probable mode of transmission of this disease was established, it became obvious that other preventive measures would be necessary to reduce transmission of this disease. One serious issue that we were forced to confront early in this epidemic was that of the bathhouses, sex clubs, and other establishments which encouraged and facilitated multiple anonymous sexual contacts. It became obvious, especially when we had a fair idea of the probable mode of transmission, that there was going to be a much greater chance of infectious contact in these facilities. There was considerable pressure in the political arena to close these establishments. I think part of that approach was shortsighted— what we were confronted with was, in reality, a behavioral disease, primarily because a person's behavior could determine, to a large extent, whether he would be exposed to the AIDS virus. We felt that in order to reduce the spread of this disease we had to effect a change in the behavior of the community as a whole. We attempted, initially, to educate those people who frequented the bathhouses. I do not feel the effort was terribly successful. We have noticed, however, that as of April, 1984, the incidence of gonorrhea had decreased by 75%. Although this is probably one of the most significant changes of behavior in the history of modern medicine, it has taken place and gone largely unnoticed. An incredible change of sexual behavior has taken place in the gay community in San Francisco and other areas.

The bathhouses continued to be a serious problem in the city until very recently. I attempted along with others to take legal and other action against the bathhouses. I felt, at the time, that if the gay community would cooperate, that a tremendous educational impact could be had on the gay and straight community. I knew that a concerned gay community could be effective in this regard because of a prior experience with an organized group of gays. In previous years in San Francisco, a number of gay bars had only one exit. Of course, this was a serious hazard in case of a fire. After much discussion with the bar owners, it became apparent that they would not comply without a significant amount of convincing of the validity of the concept. Members of the gay community formed picket lines and exerted pressure in an effort to convince the bar owners to install another exit. Several weeks later after the picket lines were established, there were two exits at all of the affected bars. Initially, I had hoped that the gay community would respond in a like manner and attempt to close the bathhouses; however, it did not choose to do so. I met with a group of federal, state, and local experts in an effort to deal with the bathhouses. The Attorney for the City of San Francisco informed us that absolute closure could not be accomplished through the courts. We discussed this and other approaches and concluded that we should establish licensure regulations. The regulations would brighten the lights in the bathhouses and make various other changes which would tend to make it unlikely that individuals would have sexual intercourse in the bathhouses. These regulations were drafted; however, for "political" reasons, it soon became obvious that the regulations would not be promulgated. The group of experts met again to discuss the various alternatives that could be taken. There were differing opinions as to what should be done. Some experts felt that any action taken to close the bathhouses would not affect the behavior of the gay community. The mayor of San Francisco, Dianne Feinstein, had said several years earlier that if the problem had been with heterosexual facilities, that I would have closed them immediately, which is true because such action would not adversely affect what we were trying to accomplish. I did not close the gay bathhouses at that time primarily because bathhouses served as a symbol to many oppressed people in San Francisco. Closing the bathhouses would only have further alienated this population, and cast the Department of Public Health in a policeman role, without creating the conditions for the essential behavioral change in the community. We had to be viewed as protectors, winning community support and assistance in trying to stem the spread of the disease.

I caused the 30 establishments in question to be evaluated, to ascertain whether high risk activities were taking place. I ordered the closure of 14 of those establishments in September, 1984. They reopened the next day. We went to court in an effort to secure a temporary restraining order. The restraining order was granted and the bathhouses were closed. After the restraining order was granted and upheld on appeal, we appeared before the judge at the preliminary injunction stage. The court modified the restraining order, allowing the bathhouses to remain open. Due to the serious public health concerns, however, the lights in the bathhouses would have to be turned up, a number of areas would have to be closed off, and there could be no sex in the bathhouses. We were quite pleased with the result; it seemed very similar to the result we wanted when we had prepared the regulations in the spring.

It is also interesting to note that when it appeared as though the bathhouses were to be closed early in spring, 1984, there were demonstrations, parades of people clad only in towels, and a great commotion over the issue. All of my mail on the issue was negative, significantly so. In October, only six months later, mail from the gay community was over 60% in favor of the closing the bathhouses. A rally against the court action in front of City Hall attracted 15 people. Only several hundred demonstrators showed up at a demonstration in the Castro area. Obviously, the public debates and discussions between April and October, as well as increasing numbers of AIDS cases, had a significant impact on the public's perception of the problem.

I was very concerned that there would be significant, adverse ramifications of any actions taken to control the spread of the disease. I feared that if we closed bathhouses in San Francisco, other, perhaps more repressive actions, would take place in other cities. Of course, we were not telling people not to have sex. We were concerned, however, that there were certain establishments where the people were profiting from the promotion, facilitation, and spread of this disease, while we were spending at that time, in San Francisco alone, $8 million to stem the spread of the disease. To allow these facilities to remain open in a commercial way, fostering the spread of the disease, did not make sense. Again, we were not telling people they could not have sex; we were just saying there were certain locations where it was not appropriate. I suppose that some people would feel that their civil liberties would be violated if we told them they could not have sex in a restaurant or a church. I think that our regulations are to be viewed in a similar way. If a person wanted to open a Russian roulette parlor, they could do so legally. They would provide the setting, the circumstances, perhaps even provide the gun with one bullet in the chamber. The patron visiting the Russian roulette parlor, not the owner, would spin the chamber of the gun. Some of the patrons would die. The same analogy holds true for the bathhouses; the law and the public support of the law has prevented such potentially lethal situations from existing.

I was at a meeting in New York City, several months ago, of gay physicians. The gay physicians obviously had opinions as to whether the bathhouses should have been closed. To those who were most adamant against the action I took, I posed this question: if there were an AIDS epidemic and there were no bathhouses, sex clubs, or other similar establishments, and there were a community effort made to open such clubs, would you want them to be opened? Not one physician in the room would say yes. I conclude, from this vote of confidence, that these physicians assume that there is at least some significant relationship between those establishments and the spread of this disease.

I have described San Francisco's full response to the AIDS crisis, and am proud to conclude that it serves as a model for the nation. Of course, other cities are trying also to meet the challenge. Significant issues still face us, however. The ensuing materials, I believe, clearly delineate some of the problems that we must address and resolve. Some of these issues include the following: when do the rights of individuals become subordinate to those of society? How do we balance social need with the AIDS victim's civil rights and liberties? Does the government have the right to close an establishment the structure of which is not inherently unsafe because it may not be in the best interest of the public health? What about prostitution? Several months ago in San Francisco, a reporter, a member of the San Francisco police department's vice squad, and a prostitute came into the public health clinic. To abuse a pun, these were strange bedfellows. They appeared at the AIDS clinic at 4:30 on a Friday, demanding that the patient (the prostitute) be seen immediately. She had not been feeling well for quite a while and it was possible that she had AIDS. Obviously, it is quite impossible to conclusively make a diagnosis of AIDS after only a physical exam. The woman's first statement was that even though she had to have the diagnosis, she would have to be out on the street to earn a living. This example poses problems that go far beyond the AIDS issue. While there may be alternatives for many people, for a number of people, including some prostitutes, there are no alternatives. If this woman is diagnosed as having AIDS, what is she going to do? She still has to feed and clothe herself, and if the only thing she can do to take care of herself is to solicit sex for money, then she will probably do so. The AIDS epidemic is made much more complex by these human tragedies.

What will be the impact on the mental health of a large and growing segment of our society as the number of AIDS patients continues to multiply? How will we meet the need for support for the friends, caretakers, and loved ones of those who are suffering and dying, not to mention the hundreds of thousands of individuals who have been told that their blood has been contaminated by HTLV-III? What role will the Food and Drug Administration play?

The screening test is a good screening test for blood; it is not a good test for people. I attempted to convince the Food and Drug Administration and the Offices of the Secretary of Health and Human Services to delay the issuance of this test until alternative testing sites could be developed. Individuals might go to a blood donation site just for the test; in so doing, they risk contaminating the blood supply. Also, I requested that there be a moratorium on giving the results to donors at these blood centers, so that we would have an opportunity to establish alternative testing sites. The FDA delayed licensing the test for approximately one month, then proceeded with the release of the test kit. Obviously, alternative testing sites were not established during that time frame. Even though I had been assured by the FDA Commissioner that there would be a moratorium on giving out the test results for at least the first three months after the test was released, a moratorium was not instituted. It seemed a blatant disregard for some of the difficult issues the test raises.

At the time of this writing, over 100 children have been diagnosed with AIDS. How will day care centers, schools, and other facilities cope with the hysteria surrounding their presence in these institutions? All of us must continue to work together to prevent the further spread of this tragic disease, and to care for its unfortunate victims.

In the late '60s and early '70s, they used to say, "If you aren't working towards the solution, then you are part of the problem." Today, unless all of us work hard to find the answers to this tragic disease, and, of equal importance, to understand the social, legal, and ethical implications of actions taken in light of AIDS, then we may actually increase the problems of AIDS in the future. I hope that these deliberations will be an important step towards addressing these important issues.

Government Involvement and the Development of Public Policy in AIDS Research and Reporting

Edward N. Brandt, Jr., M.D., Ph.D.
Chancellor, The University of Maryland
Former Assistant Secretary for Health
Department of Health and Human Services

AIDS is an extremely complex scientific entity. It destroys the immune system of its victims. It is uniformly fatal. Over 10,000 Americans have contracted this disease; over 4,000 of these Americans have died. We heard about the first three cases of AIDS in 1981 from UCLA, and then an additional two cases appeared. Since that time, millions of dollars, a great deal of thought, and a lot of work have been spent in an attempt to understand and control this disease and to care for those persons who are afflicted by it. Fortunately, in recent years it has attracted the attention of some of the finest minds in American science. Considering the complexity of the illness, significant scientific progress has been made. I had the opportunity to attend a portion of the International Conference on AIDS in spring, 1985 and was overwhelmed by efforts being expended and the progress being made to understand this disorder. At the same time, however, major sociopolitical issues have been raised, largely revolving around the two groups of people who early on were at greatest risk of developing AIDS.

Because of the complexity of the disease, and because of the sociopolitical overtones, even standard epidemic control measures, such as surveillance, had to be thoroughly reexamined. It is clear that many persons afflicted with this disease, or at high risk for it, are also subject to social, political, and legal risks. In my view, if one considers that AIDS was unknown at the time it was first observed, that it is scientifically complex, that it renders its victims incapable of disease resistance, that it occurs largely in people around whom swirls significant social controversies, then AIDS represents a unique epidemic in our history.

I would like to share with you, in a somewhat objective fashion, some of my thoughts about various social, political, ethical, and public policy issues. The first and, in my opinion, one of the most vexing issues that has been raised in this epidemic, is that of confidentiality. When investigating an epidemic it is helpful, and in fact almost essential, to be able to trace individuals, their exposures, contacts, and the nature of those contacts with other people. It is difficult to investigate thoroughly an epidemic without access to names or other identifying information. With AIDS, however, we are faced with the fact that disclosure of this information puts people afflicted with the disease at other risks. These considerations lead to a real dilemma. Do we sacrifice the completeness of our epidemiologic studies to protect the rights of the suffering, or do we somehow adopt the maxim that the rights of the many outweigh those of the few? Furthermore, if a government agency was not collecting these epidemiologic data, would it be less likely that the data would be revealed or publicly scrutinized? Perhaps the correct answer lies somewhere in between, assuming that there is a right answer. At present, our current approach to gathering information about AIDS is done in the same fashion as any other infectious sexually transmitted disease, whether the data are gathered by city health departments, county health departments, state health departments, or the federal government through the Centers for Disease Control. I maintain, however, based on my experience, that there are no secrets in government. There is no assurance of individual privacy at any level of government, especially at the federal level. Government records are public documents for all intents and purposes. Although those of us in the Public Health Service (PHS) insisted consistently that we would protect the confidentiality of the people being studied, the media, congressional staff, and potentially even private citizens will most probably have little impediment to gaining access to those records. As some of you know who attended a recent, well-publicized hearing, there was a direct confrontation between the PHS and the Congress over these issues. In my opinion, the problems related to lack of confidentiality of medical and other information and the balancing social necessity of thoroughly investigating this epidemic requires very careful analysis. It should not be necessary to put people at risk of invasion of privacy in order to protect other people. Whether this requires legislation, as has been proposed by a number of groups, or whether other means are indicated, is not clear to me. I think it does deserve careful evaluation, however, and the careful drafting of a clear statement of any solution to the problem.

The second important issue, in my view, is definition of the roles of the various parties that have a responsibility to investigate and potentially develop solutions to problems such as AIDS. There needs to be a clearer understanding of the roles to be played by local health departments, state health departments, and the federal government. In the case of a geographically confined epidemic, these roles appear to be obvious, and that, of course, is generally the approach adopted. Early in the epidemic of AIDS there were two cities primarily involved, namely, New York and San Francisco. The country was very fortunate that those two cities had health department leadership of excellent quality that could and did respond in a truly outstanding fashion. I stand in awe of them. At the same time, however, we cannot expect all local health departments to possess the expertise that is required to address the problems that will arise with patients with AIDS. It is simply too expensive, even if the people who are trained to address this sort of disease were available. The natural place to find such expertise, in most people's view, is in the federal government. I do not believe it is the only place. Universities are a significant source of such experts, and their expertise can be tapped through a number of arrangements to examine epidemics and advise health officials. Indeed, the Centers for Disease Control (CDC) is very much dependent on a group of people known as Epidemic Intelligence Service (EIS) officers, experts in the specific epidemic confronting them. The role of this and other groups should be reexamined especially when rights and obligations are in conflict. In certain aspects of epidemic control, for example, local health departments maintain the sovereign power to close businesses. These powers are derived from the police powers of the state, not from the federal government. The best example of this in the AIDS epidemic, of course, was the issue of closing the bathhouses. Irrespective of individual rights concerns, there is still an issue as to whether the federal government had the authority to close bathhouses under any circumstances. Furthermore, it was not possible for those of us in Washington to determine, in every locale in the United States, whether closing the bathhouses would have any impact on AIDS in that particular area. In our view, that decision could be made only by local health officials. Thus, we decided that we did not have the authority to close bathhouses, or prevent any other legitimate business concern from operating, even though a particular concern may have been considered by the media or other groups to be a significant public health problem. Further, we did not know whether such closings would accomplish anything even if we could have done it.

The third issue relates to general public health policy matters. In my view, the major public health policy concerns about AIDS should be addressed including the necessity for an adequate detection system, a good surveillance system, prompt response capabilities, adequate mechanisms for public information, central coordination of scientific effort, and a clear definition of the roles of the various participants. It is clear that we can learn a great deal about the adequacies and inadequacies of our current health policies from this epidemic. A reevaluation of these issues should occur in an objective fashion and outside the current partisan political debate over AIDS.

Another policy issue that deserves our more immediate attention relates to the provision of medical care to persons afflicted by a disastrous epidemic like AIDS. In one sense, this can be considered a part of the general problem of uncompensated care in this country. It can also be looked upon, however, as part of a disaster response planning system. Certainly, tornadoes, hurricanes, earthquakes, and similar events can produce large numbers of victims requiring intensive and expensive care, who may not have third-party payment sources for such injuries. Across the United States, the various states and jurisdictions approach these problems in different ways. Some states approach the problem on a county, city, or other local level; other states address care issues through more central control. Also, there are a number of federal programs including Medicaid, Medicare and its disability program, block grants, and perhaps even disaster aid that can be utilized. I claim no special expertise in this area; however, I believe that the situation deserves the attention of persons with the knowledge, expertise, and ability to address these cost issues. I recommend that the various parties involved, including the governors' association, the mayors' association, state and territorial health officers, city and county health officials, the federal government, and other interested parties meet to address these issues. As I recount the list of people who clearly have a role and an interest in this problem, you will note that I am rapidly approaching the seating capacity of Boston's Fenway Park. Therefore, these groups should meet to first decide how to solve the problem, rather than first trying to solve the problem. An intelligent plan that takes into account the varying responsibilities, legal and otherwise, shared by all of these officials, could be developed and is essential.

The three topics that have aroused the greatest debate during this period include the scientific response to the epidemic, the funding of same, and the blood test for antibodies to HTLV-III (or LAV, depending on your nationality). Because of my personal involvement in these issues, I apologize in advance for any lack of objectivity that is apparent; however, I have had an opportunity to give these matters some thought outside of the political arena, and have gained some insight, I think, through discussions with various people concerned with AIDS. Now that I no longer have any responsibility to provide researchers with funds, they can be somewhat more candid; on the other hand, so can I.

Scientific response to the AIDS epidemic was criticized quite heavily early in the effort, and to some extent, is still being criticized. When we considered the scientific steps that would be necessary to fight this epidemic in 1981 and early in 1982, we had to adopt some major principles. These principles included the following:

1. AIDS is a scientifically complex disease;

2. we could not afford to sponsor mediocre, poor or otherwise misleading scientific research, since the results of such research could or would raise false hopes and frustrate constructive effort;

3. we would adhere to the proven system of strict peer review of all research;

4. we would integrate the AIDS scientific efforts into the overall scientific efforts of the Public Health Service, since we felt that many of those other efforts might contribute to gaining insight into AIDS; and

5. we would mobilize the internal scientific capabilities of the Public Health Service, especially those at the CDC and the National Institutes of Health (NIH), to investigate this epidemic.

In addition to these principles, we were determined to seek the widest possible advice from scientists. The most controversial decision of all was to resist any efforts to alter our scientific approach on the basis of political or public relations expediency. Scientific progress does not occur by leapfrogging from breakthrough to breakthrough; rather, it occurs by carefully and meticulously moving step by step towards the scientific solution of a problem. I hope that few people will disagree that the discovery of HTLV-III as an etiologic factor in AIDS was a major step. Indeed, as I look back over the great epidemics that have struck man, I know of no other example where so much progress was made in so short a time. This discovery was based also upon a great deal of work. Early studies by series of investigators had narrowed the search for an etiologic agent down to a virus. Early efforts with isolation led to the suspicion that a retrovirus might be involved, although at that time only one other known human disease due to a retrovirus had ever been described. That retrovirus, of course, is responsible for the development of T-cell leukemia/lymphoma. Since the discovery of HTLV-III, scientific efforts have mushroomed. Virtually all aspects of the functioning of the immune system, the biology of retroviruses, the management of complications of AIDS, and even the development of antiviral agents have grown exponentially. I believe that all of mankind will benefit for many, many years from the research that has been completed and is underway in addressing AIDS.

The benefits of central coordination of AIDS research, in my opinion, helped. Early on, a committee was created and designed to share scientific information. I am now convinced, however, that a more detailed assignment of responsibilities and sharing of results would have been even more beneficial. Would that have sped up the results? I do not believe so; however, I think it would have given greater assurance to the scientific community, and to the public, had our efforts appeared more systematic. I also believe that at an appropriate time it would be desirable to reexamine this nation's ability to implement a scientific response to major epidemics. The basic mission of the National Institutes of Health and other scientific granting institutions is to develop medical science, with the goal of gaining further insight into human biology, human health, and human disease. We must be cautious not to cause the scientific community to address every outbreak of disease that arises, to the expense of these scientists' basic research foci. The natural selection of research efforts has led, in the past, to unexpected scientific advances. The reorientation of research priorities requires careful evaluation through peer review. On the other hand, the acceleration of the peer review process and other steps that were taken by the NIH to expedite research funding should be studied with an eye towards having such a mechanism in place so that it can be called upon when the situation warrants it. This should also apply to the publication of scientific articles. I believe the major scientific journals of the country responded in a most effective way to expedite their peer review, and by permitting the release of scientific findings following acceptance of research, but prior to publication. Again, I would emphasize that peer review in this process must be preserved, or we will simply have confusion, anxiety, and panic.

The funding of the efforts to solve the AIDS tragedy is the most contentious of all of the controversies surrounding AIDS. It has been mixed with partisan political efforts and has included some rather severe personal attacks. My own judgment is that the controversy over funding has detracted from the scientific efforts and contributed greatly to confusion in the public's mind. Partisan political statements attract the media and can quickly destroy the credibility of good science. At the same time, however, I recognize that in any republic based on democratic principles, such political controversies are a way of life. I accept them because the alternative is simply too great a price to pay. One of the things that shocked me when I came to Washington was that scientific efforts in Washington are largely evaluated on the amount of money spent on them, rather than on their results. It seems axiomatic to me that research in certain areas will cost less money than research in others. Consider, as a example, the cost of research in new imaging techniques using devices like the PET scanner, the MRI, and so forth, as compared to research on the mechanism of action of certain enzymes. Yet we continue to compare apples to oranges in the funding business. The basic issue is, should more money have been spent on research in AIDS? Would it have moved the progress any faster? I think it is still too early to tell for certain. I continue to believe that during the first three years of this epidemic we had enough money to deal with the scientific aspects of this disease in a rational, thoughtful, and orderly fashion. There is no question that we could have spent more money. The Public Health Service is very good at spending money. But I would point out to you that we were funding research proposals with a priority score considerably lower than that which would have been funded at any other time during the history of the NIH in order to spend the money that we had at the time. That concerned me because I firmly believe that mediocre research results in more harm than good. At no time did I ever prevent or influence the Public Health Service agencies from requesting what they believed to be necessary funds. Their requests were not altered by me in any way. Further, I am convinced that our requests for funding for AIDS research were based upon the most reasonable course of action to be followed that we could identify at the time.

There are two misconceptions that I believe need clarification. The first of these has to do with the reprogramming of funds. The budgetary system of the federal government is somewhat complex; frankly, no one understands it. When an agency attempts to allocate or request funding for an issue such as AIDS or any other nonpredictable problem, it is markedly easier and faster to reprogram excess funds from one established program into the nonpredictable funding problem area. Those excess funds would ordinarily lapse back into the Treasury and supplemental appropriations would have to be requested. In all instances, we reprogrammed funds that were clearly at excess, that would have lapsed into the Treasury under any circumstances and had already been so designated, and applied them to the AIDS area. From a symbolic, and I expect from a public relations point of view, it would have been better to have lapsed the funds, and requested supplemental appropriations. It would have been considerably slower, however, and resulted in even further delays and debate.

The second area which should be clarified relates to the redirection of the internal efforts of the Public Health Service. In every emergent problem about which I am aware, it was necessary to consult with and gather the necessary expertise to address a given problem. During the past four years, we have had a number of rather serious issues arise. A few of those issues include the Tylenol tragedy, where we had, within 24 hours, hundreds of people working to address, contain, and solve that problem; the issue of the safety of vaccines; also, a number of environmental issues arose, such as Times Beach, Love Canal, and others. In each of these instances, we utilized the expertise of the Public Health Service to address those problems. Clearly, these experts were redirected from what they were doing otherwise. It is simply not possible to bring in outside expertise quickly enough, given the exigencies of relocating people and going through the federal personnel system. Although it would be worthwhile for the scientific community and the Public Health Service to examine this process of internal redirection, and perhaps to define alternatives, my own view, from having been subjected to it for four years, is that it is probably not all that bad.

Finally, let me address relevant issues relating to the blood test. At the time of the discovery of HTLV-III and the ELISA (enzyme-linked immunosorbent assay) test to detect antibodies to the virus, we were confronted with two significant problems. The first problem related to the quality of the supply of blood available for transfusions. The second problem involved trying to define the natural history and detailed epidemiology of AIDS. Both of these were clearly hampered by our inability to recognize the presence of either infection or exposure. The blood test presented the first step forward in addressing both of these problems. I am fully aware of and sympathetic with the fact that the blood test presented then, and presents now, a dramatic potential for abuse and misuse. In many ways it is a classic clash. We had the opportunity to identify blood that could put the recipient at risk of AIDS. However, we had the potential to develop a list of people who had positive tests, putting them at a great societal risk. Finally, we had the problem of interpreting the implications of a positive test to those people who test positive to the antibody. It seems to me that the current policy of establishing alternative testing sites might be the best solution, under the circumstances, to protect the blood supply. The possibility of high risk individuals donating blood in order to obtain the blood test results is a very real threat to the viability of our blood supply.

Further, the problem of confidentiality of these results raises serious issues. The possibility of preventing AIDS infections through the use of transfused blood is a lifesaving measure. Despite the false-negative and false-positive results that occasionally result, the potential for saving lives still remains. It would be better if we had a more exact test. It would be better if the test would be useful in diagnosis as well as in detecting antibodies to the virus. Unfortunately, we do not have such a test, and we have to use a test with limited utility. Its primary utility remains in the area of removing contaminated blood from our blood banks. Second, it may help us in understanding the early phases of this disease. I am convinced that something can be done about the disease through early intervention; however, we do not know what this something is yet.

It is clearly essential that we take the time to study this epidemic from every perspective and in great detail. We are a nation with diverse views on social, religious, and health issues. There will be disagreements; difficult decisions must be made. As time passes and we put these issues into some perspective, we will learn a great deal through the consideration and resolution of the various social and public policy issues that have been raised by AIDS. If we ever have another disaster like AIDS hit this country, I hope that history will find us much better prepared.

Question

(Michael Callen): My personal experience contradicts your funding presentation. I am a member of one of the first and longest prospective studies on AIDS. At many points in the early days of that study it was almost discontinued for lack of funds. Other studies were similarly short of funding from any source. Also, at the spring, 1985 hearing in Washington, a week after you testified that $17 million was sufficient, and that you could hardly spend that amount, you then more than doubled your funding request. Was that only a political dance? Did you genuinely believe that the funding requested by the Department was adequate and that only because of our lobbying efforts you asked for more money than was needed?

Answer

I think that I remember the hearing somewhat better than you do. In many ways, the testimony marked a turning point in the controversy. I still believe that we had sufficient funds. Frankly, I remember some testimony before the Congress, by various people, who said that they were unable to get their grants funded. When we evaluated those requests further, however, we found that we had not received funding applications from those people. The Public Health Service is not in the habit of sending money to people and then asking for an application. I maintain that we had sufficient funds at the time of the hearing to support first-class research into this problem. Some of the research that we were funding was not as sophisticated as it should have been, given the exigencies of this crisis. We were very optimistic that additional research projects would be forthcoming; we did, in fact, exercise a reasonable amount of generosity in our requests. We were not trying to play a political game. Also, I never discouraged any efforts to educate Congress about the issues. Perhaps your groups were effective in helping to ensure that adequate funding was made available. We could have spent more money; I do not think that we could have done so wisely.

Balancing Individual and Societal Rights

Sheldon Landesman, M.D.
Associate Professor of Medicine
Downstate Medical Center
Director, AIDS Study Group

It is clear that the acquired immune deficiency syndrome, or AIDS, is a unique medical disease, and has given rise to a unique set of moral, ethical, and legal problems. In exploring these problems, however, one must explore the known facts of the disease, determine how they are unique, and how they give rise to the derivative social, legal, and ethical issues.

The newly described HTLV-III virus is the cause of AIDS. The disease itself is just one part of a series of potential outcomes for a person with an HTLV-III infection. The number of HTLV-III infected individuals is far greater than the number of persons who have AIDS. I believe that the most thorny problems will arise when society attempts to handle presently healthy persons who are infected with HTLV-III.

The HTLV-III virus is related closely to a variety of viruses that cause chronic, latent, long-term infections in animals, and have chronic sequelae, such as neurological disease or chronic pulmonary disease. Some of the chronic long-term effects seen with these animal viruses also represent possible outcomes for individuals infected with HTLV-III.

In modern times, we have not encountered a disease with the propensity and power that this virus has to cause disease. The only real analogy that I can think of is that of syphilis in the 16th century when it was first introduced into Europe. Like the syphilis spirochete, HTLV-III is a blood and venereally transmitted, potentially lethal infectious disease. Unlike the syphilis spirochete, the incubation period from exposure to serious injury from this virus is measured in years, as opposed to decades. Evidence now strongly suggests that the infection is chronic, if not lifelong. The infection may be communicable even when an infected person is asymptomatic, which means that it is not easy to clinically identify a person who carries the virus and, therefore, may transmit it. Only by performing HTLV-III testing can a healthy infected individual be identified. The single most important factor here is that there is a high correlation between an

HTLV-III antibody test positive and the presence of the virus. Based upon the scientific evidence that we now have in hand, those persons with antibody positivity are presumptively virus positive, and therefore at risk of transmitting the disease to other persons.

The total number of HTLV-III positive persons is estimated between 700,000 and one million; thus, it appears that there is an enormously large pool of persons, ranging from the asymptomatic, antibody and virus positive persons, to others with milder manifestations of HTLV-III infection, in our society. It is important to remember that these people are at least potentially infectious (via blood, sexual contact, or mother to offspring) to other persons. How to deal with these persons in a manner that is both consistent with their civil rights and consistent with the public health needs of other citizens is the issue. There are legitimate but very conflicting priorities and claims in relationship to the prevention of the spread of this disease versus civil liberties. How we resolve those conflicting but legitimate claims is going to be a measure of our society's sensitivity and ability to deal with complex social issues. As the debate heats up over the next several years, it is important to remember that we should listen to one another, that there are going to be people who have views or put forth arguments which may be diametrically opposed to the arguments of other persons, and, yet, they may be equally legitimate. If we do not listen to each other in this debate, then the final outcome through societal notions, mores, and rules may be much worse than anticipated.

One serious issue before us is in the area of the individual's responsibility to society, to friends, and to sexual contacts. What do you do if you are an HTLV-III positive person, are young, and are sexually active? Is it your responsibility to tell your sexual mates that you are HTLV-III antibody positive and therefore potentially infectious to them? Is it your individual decision to decide to refrain from sexual contact and therefore deny yourself what is obviously one of life's very normal pleasures? This sort of decision will be made by individuals in a very private and personal manner. How this decision is made, however, will very much be influenced by societal views towards these individuals. If they are treated with a certain degree of gentleness and understanding, then it may be possible for them to make better decisions in a more enlightened and reasonable light. If they are treated as members of the greater community they will respond as such. If they are treated as social outcasts their response is less predictable.

In light of the concerns about HTLV-III positivity, should a person seek HTLV-III testing? This question has been raised in numerous settings since the test was licensed. Some blood donors (all blood donors are now routinely tested) say that they do not want to know the results of the test. This is a profound, yet not irrational, response. They do not want to be faced with having to have to refrain from sex or feeling guilty about infecting a sexual partner. How should a person resolve the decision of whether they should be tested? If you asked people in our medical center if they want to know if they are HTLV-III test positive, many of them have and would say, "No, I don't want to know." If you ask them another question, a different response is elicited: "If you had an infectious disease that you could transmit to your wife, to your life-partner, or to your child, would you want to know now if there was a possibility that you could take action to prevent yourself from transmitting it?" Invariably, the answer to this question is "Yes." These questions outline clearly the moral dilemma that many persons are facing at the present time.

Premarital testing is an issue that is going to come up fairly soon in our society, and perhaps in New York City within the next few years. There are, at present, many thousands of heterosexual persons who are HTLV-III positive. The persons are either drug addicts or the sexual partners of addicts. All of these persons are a reservoir for the further sexual spread of virus into the heterosexual community. The women who are infected are also at significant risk of passing the virus on to their children. The question of premarital testing, as with syphilis, will be one public health response to this aspect of the disease.

The use of this test in the military is another example of the problem posed by HTLV-III infection. The United States Army at the present time has implemented mandatory HTLV-III testing for all persons to be inducted into the Army. They have also recently mandated testing for all present members in the military. Obviously, this is a complex issue. Is the military using the test to screen for and identify homosexual inductees and members of the Armed Services? Is testing a valid measure of capabilities as a soldier? Is it important to screen for HTLV-III in this setting? One concern is that HTLV-III positive persons in the military may be sent to many different countries. The military personnel may then spread the HTLV-III to prostitutes all over the world, who may infect other transient or local populations. Other soldiers without the infection may likewise become infected. It is a very relevant and difficult issue as to whether the United States government should attempt to prevent the military from exporting the disease to countries where it does not exist at present.

Another serious issue is the question of HTLV-III positive children. It is clear from preliminary scientific data that there are children who are positive carriers for the virus, are not symptomatic, and do not have the disease. Who should have access to knowledge of the HTLV-III carrier state of a particular child? If it is known that a child is HTLV-III positive, you can be fairly sure that most other parents, out of legitimate concern, will want to keep their children separated from the HTLV-III positive child. One would certainly fear the idea of establishing day care centers or separate schools for only HTLV-III positive children. I think we will have to confront this question very soon. We have a case in our hospital at the present time of a child who was born of an HTLV-III positive woman who subsequently died of AIDS. The father was unknown and could not be found. The child was kept in the hospital while awaiting placement. It was discovered that the child was HTLV-III antibody positive. The child has been kept in the hospital for over a year because no facilities are willing to take the child. In addition, the nursing staff, who are normally very loving and very caring for children in the hospital, are very reluctant to pick up the baby, to care for, handle, talk, or interact with the baby. As a result, the child has been in the hospital for a year yet has had minimal social stimulation. One day, someone brought a Cabbage Patch doll for the child and placed it on the chair next to the child. Unfortunately, it was difficult to ascertain which was the child and which was the Cabbage Patch doll. This is simply one example of the consequences of the HTLV-III epidemic that we now face; I hope that we will be able to develop a sense of how to approach these sorts of problems.

References

1. Curran, James W. 1985. The epidemiology and prevention of the acquired immunodeficiency syndrome. *Annals of Internal Medicine* 103:657–662.
2. Biggar, Robert J., B. Johnson, P. Gigase, et al. 1985. Seroepidemiology of HTLV-III in Eastern Zaire and Kenya. Paper presented at the International Conference on Acquired Immunodeficiency Syndrome, April 14–17, Atlanta, Georgia.
3. Essex, M., J. Allan, P. Kanki, et al. 1985. Antigens of human T-lymphotrophic virus type III/lymphadenopathy-associated virus. *Annals of Internal Medicine* 103:700–703.
4. Centers for Disease Control. 1985. Revision of the case definition of acquired immunodeficiency syndrome for national reporting—United States. *Morbidity and Mortality Weekly Report*. 34:373–375.
5. Centers for Disease Control. 1985. *Acquired Immunodeficiency Syndrome (AIDS) Weekly Surveillance Report—United States AIDS Activity.* September 2.
6. Lawrence, Dale N., K.-J. Lui, D.J. Bregman, et al. 1985. A model-based estimate of the average incubation and latency period for transfusion-associated AIDS. Paper presented at the International Conference on Acquired Immunodeficiency Syndrome, April 14–17, Atlanta, Georgia.

PART III
The Complications of AIDS Research

Placebo-Controlled, Double-Blind Research on Patients with AIDS

Martin S. Hirsch, M.D.
Associate Professor of Medicine, Harvard Medical School
Associate Physician, The Massachusetts General Hospital

I would like to address an issue that will become extremely important as our research progresses to the point of evaluating therapeutic modalities in patients with AIDS and AIDS-related conditions. This issue relates to the evaluation of drugs using the double-blind, placebo-controlled clinical trial. Several historical examples may be useful to illustrate the concerns.

Another virus epidemic was devastating in this country in the 1950s, namely, polio. The polio epidemic affected and crippled thousands of individuals. Over 1.8 million children were enrolled in a double-blind placebo-controlled clinical trial of the Salk polio vaccine, the results of which were announced in 1955. The participants included children from the first to the third grade; it was decided that while one grade would get the vaccine, another grade would get a placebo, and a third grade would be observed without either placebo or the vaccine.[1] No one knew who was getting the placebo or who was getting the vaccine. The results were unequivocal, demonstrating the great benefits of polio vaccination. As a result, paralytic polio has been virtually eradicated from the United States.

Another analogous situation arose in the 1960s with the disease called herpes simplex encephalitis, a disease of the brain with a mortality rate of approximately 80%. Less than 10% of affected individuals survived without brain damage. At that time, certain groups of researchers published data purporting to show that a drug called idoxuridine was effective in treating herpes encephalitis. This information was spread among clinicians who had experience with patients having herpes encephalitis. Some of us felt that the data were not convincing, and that a placebo-controlled trial needed to be done to evaluate whether the drug, in fact, was effective. We met with considerable opposition. Some of our colleagues argued that it was unethical to deny a potentially lifesaving drug to people suffering from a life-threatening disease. Despite these concerns, we proceeded with controlled trials and showed that idoxuridine was neither safe nor effective.[2] In fact, people who were treated with it did more poorly than those who were receiving the placebo. In the 1970s and 1980s, the same kind of placebo-controlled trials were used to study other anti-herpes drugs to determine whether they are effective and safe.[3] As a result of these studies, we now have drugs available that reduce the mortality of herpes encephalitis to approximately 20% to 30%.

In light of these historical precedents, we must be wary of anecdotal case reports, particularly in an infection, such as AIDS, with a long incubation period, an extended period of illness, and a variable natural history. If there is no accepted therapy, placebo controls are a necessary part of any therapeutic study. Without adequate controls, the results that are presented and often published lack validity; anecdotal reports will mislead investigators, physicians, and patients alike. Further, they may impede the development of other new drugs that may be effective.

A great deal of discussion is taking place in the press and in the scientific literature about agents that purport to be active against HTLV-III, including azidothymidine, suramin, HPA-23, ribavirin, interferon-alpha, and others. Stories have arisen that some of these agents are good, some of these agents are dangerous, some of these agents don't work. The discussions about whether these medications are good, bad or indifferent for patients with AIDS are not substantiated at the present time. Once investigators become persuaded that a medication is efficacious on scientifically invalid grounds, they may mistakenly consider themselves to be ethically bound to act and treat patients in light of these assumptions. The result is that we are often left with dangerous or ineffective agents while we discard other potentially useful agents.

With respect to HTLV-III infection, it is remarkable that in the past year, a large number of different agents have been developed that have activity against this virus in tissue cultures. A number of studies about these agents have been funded. At the time of this conference, however, only one of these agents, interferon-alpha, is currently in a multicenter, collaborative double-blind, placebo-controlled trial. We have found that in these studies, once the subjects are adequately informed about the necessity of a placebo-controlled trial, we have had little difficulty in enrolling subjects. Obviously, no one wants to take a placebo. However, if we inform patients that this is the only way that we can achieve data that will be valuable to themselves and to the community, they are more willing to proceed. Of course, we promise the participants that at the conclusion of these studies, if interferon is found to be useful, they will not be denied interferon in subsequent treatment. Other drugs are in earlier stages of development; ribavirin, suramin, HPA-23, phosphonofurmate, and azidothymidine are all agents that are in preliminary trials. I do not think that anyone should be misled—there is no evidence at the present time that any of these medications is beneficial for patients with AIDS. Only with carefully controlled trials will we be able to evaluate whether they do or do not help these patients.

It is important to realize that the goals of medical scientists working on AIDS are the same as those of the people afflicted with the disease; that is, to end the suffering and misery associated with the disease. The quickest way to control AIDS is through validly conducted and carefully controlled clinical trials. Shortcuts will not work.

Controlled Therapeutic Trials on Patients with AIDS

Clyde Crumpacker, M.D.

Associate Professor of Medicine, Harvard Medical School

Department of Infectious Diseases, Beth Israel Hospital

The ethical commitment of physicians and health care providers to do what they can to help patients frequently conflicts with the careful, scientific approach to medicine. They even appear, on occasion, to be taking contradictory approaches. Perhaps the disease of AIDS heightens the dilemmas associated with AIDS research because of the overwhelming desire to help the afflicted, dying patient. The dilemma that we face, though, is not really a new one. Francis Peabody, the founder of the Thorndike Laboratory at Boston City Hospital, observed in the 1927 Gay lecture on Medical Ethics that there is no more contradiction between the science of medicine and the art of healing than between the science of aviation and the art of flying.[4] This statement accents an ideal that we all strive to achieve. I think Dr. Peabody realized the potential tension between caring for patients and the best way to achieve this care. Dr. Peabody also stated that the secret of the care of the patient is caring for the patient.[4] An excellent example of ethical medicine is in the trial of the hepatitis B vaccine in the high risk gay male population in New York City. There were over 1,000 participants in the trial, and it was meticulously designed and carried out as a placebo-controlled trial.[5] The rigorous science was matched by the tremendous courage and dedication of all the participants. The cooperation and involvement of the participants and the gay community in New York represented a milestone of participation, with people doing everything they could to make sure the science would be as impeccable as possible. Since the vaccine was found to be effective, in as expeditious a manner as possible through the double-blind approach, the vaccine is now available to everyone. The real scientific dilemma would have been raised if the researchers had failed to perform a careful study and were uncertain as to whether the vaccine would be effective. A double-blind trial is the only method available, at present, that screens researcher, subject, and other potential biases from affecting the results. The decision not to perform such a trial may waste inordinate amounts of time and energy and may jeopardize the health of a patient subjected to a treatment that is not efficacious.

As a recent example of the importance of these carefully conducted clinical trials, at the Beth Israel and Brigham and Women's Hospital, I have been involved in a study of interferon as a potential treatment in bone marrow transplant recipients. When people undergo bone marrow transplantation, their marrow's capacity to create new cells is destroyed by irradiation, in order to allow the bone marrow graft to be effective. These patients become infected readily with different viruses, in some ways similar to patients with AIDS. Interferon is being evaluated in an attempt to prevent these viral infections. One patient in the study had done very well. She had no infections and was discharged from the hospital in a minimal amount of time. We were all convinced that interferon was wonderful. When we looked at the patient code for the double-blind trial, we discovered to our surprise that she had been getting a placebo and not the interferon. Perhaps we did her a favor by not giving her the interferon—perhaps it may have made her ill had she received it. Thus, there really is no replacement for a carefully performed scientific trial.

In addition to the double-blind trials which are underway, there is a need for compassionate plea trials. Compassionate plea trials usually occur in the setting where there is no therapy available, when we really do not know what to do, and we have a drug that perhaps could do something. On a historical basis, little is ever learned from these compassionate plea trials because it is very difficult to locate and evaluate the records. Treatment is usually rendered in a desperate situation, with therapy given when there are many confounding factors. It is very hard to sort out whether the particular therapy has been helpful or whether apparent benefits are fortuitous. The therapy may even be harmful, making things worse than they were without the therapy. Two very well-known examples exist where this nonscientific approach to evaluating therapy is proceeding at present. The artificial heart program will most likely never be evaluated through a controlled trial because of the use of this rationale for justifying untested therapies. Another example is the use of antibiotics in open heart surgery. It has never been submitted to a controlled trial to test whether antibiotics, in general, or which antibiotics minimize infections following heart surgery. Every surgeon in the world uses these antibiotics. It would be unrealistic to think that a placebo-controlled trial would be considered or attempted, given the gravity of the risk of infection.

Because of the problems that these patients face, research is only one element of the total support system that is necessary. The research team has to collaborate closely with the support workers, keeping in mind that a research trial is not therapy. It is an experiment that hopefully will identify a treatment.

An additional factor in research is the need for the research to be carried out in a strongly supportive setting. The research team should interact closely with the support team of health care professionals in treating patients with AIDS.

On occasion, the study protocol may appear to conflict with a need to treat a study participant. For example, if a patient is in a double-blind trial and develops pneumonia, could the study therapy be exacerbating pneumonia? Whenever these questions arise, the research and health care teams have to be willing to put the protocols aside. The care of the patient must be first and foremost. If the protocol code has to be entered to find out what drug the patient is getting, then the study must be secondary.

Lastly, the research in this area must be associated with a commitment to education. Researchers are always closest to the new data and the new findings. They may understand that a medication or technique is going to work before other members of the health care team. This perspective needs to be shared, as soon as possible, with all the members of the health care team, through publications and lectures. Only through the dogged persistence of the researchers and tenacious adherence to careful scientific principles will we develop a solution to this disease.

Comment

Despite the positive aspects of performing placebo-controlled clinical trials, there may be some opposition to performing them. For example, in the polio vaccine trial, the justification for having a placebo group at the outset was that there simply was not enough vaccine to go around. The researchers knew there would be a large number of children who would not receive vaccine so they decided to distribute this by random allocation. This is one way of circumventing some of the protests about withholding a treatment when you have reasonable grounds to suspect that it might be useful.

We heard about the idoxuridine trial for herpes simplex encephalitis. A decade later, when there was a similar trial for the use of ara-A in herpes simplex encephalitis, a very heated controversy was generated. In general, there is a problem with the withholding of active therapy when you have some cause to suspect it will be helpful, especially when it is active therapy, designed to mitigate the disabling or lethal components of a disease.

Another example relates to the randomized clinical trials that revealed how corticosteroids were both harmful and useless in the treatment of children with rheumatic fever. The person who established these trials was branded a murderer in an editorial in the professional journal of his own specialty. These studies evoke powerful emotion and most probably will continue to do so.

Question

I agree with Dr. Hirsch that controlled clinical trials in the use of antiviral agents and other possible treatment of AIDS are absolutely essential. I differ somewhat, however, in that they need to be placebo-controlled. In this particular instance, historical controls—meaning people who in the past were diagnosed with AIDS and were not treated with these substances—could be used, instead of placebos. If you have a sufficiently large "pool" of patients to draw from, and if those historical controls are sufficiently similar and can be matched for severity of disease, for natural history, for age, and for whatever other characteristics may determine the cause, then historical controls could in fact, be valid comparisons.

Historical controls in the past have been the subject of derision because the controls often were not comparable. For instance, in various forms of heart disease, tremendous medical successes have occurred in treating arrhythmias. We have some experience with useful treatments of arrhythmias, both in the past and in the present. However, persons with AIDS have, for all intents and purposes, been given no treatment at all. We have a disease that is almost certainly fatal; we are running a very great ethical risk in giving a patient a placebo; in so doing, we are denying possibly effective treatments to people who face certain death otherwise. I would rather use historical controls.

Answer

(Robert J. Levine, M.D.): These concerns have been raised in a number of other situations in the past, including herpes simplex encephalitis. Another situation where the concern was raised was in the area of the disease osteosarcoma. About ten years ago, interferon was claimed to be very efficacious when compared to historical controls. Through a placebo-controlled trial, this was discovered not to be the case.

Let me suggest, though, that one of the landmark events in what we now see as research ethics was the publication in 1970 of *Experimentation with Human Subjects* edited by Paul A. Freund.[6] In one chapter, David Rudstein of Harvard Medical School identified one area in which his statement has been since treated as noncontroversial. That is, if you had a disease that was uniformly lethal, that it would be unethical to do a placebo-controlled trial. He gave as this example, rabies: if you had a drug that on theoretical grounds might bring about a cure or a remission in a patient with rabies, then it would be unethical to set up a placebo-control study. I propose that if we accept Dr. Rudstein's notion, we would not now know that idoxuridine is neither effective nor safe in the treatment of herpes encephalitis. The natural history of HTLV-III infection is still under study. We know that people can survive for long periods of time. I would agree with Dr. Crumpacker in that early treatment is important, not only early in the development of disease, but also early in the course of infection. A patient dying from AIDS probably should not be given a placebo. Of the more likely beneficial results of treatment with the present candidates for therapy, results will most likely be seen in patients early in their course of infection. In that setting, if you rely on historical controls, or if you do not perform placebo-controlled trials, you will not produce reliable data as you may miss an early beneficial result.

Comment

Because medicine is advancing so rapidly in this area, I also am not convinced that historical controls are sufficient. Our abilities to treat the disease and its severe manifestations are changing dramatically. For example, respirator technology is improving, and different combinations of drugs for treating infections are continually evolving. Some of the techniques we are using now we were not even thinking about three months ago. The interferon example is a good one—should we give everyone interferon? Interferon operates on many different levels. It is a very effective cell stimulator; it may also be toxic. Without a control group, the harmful effects would not be apparent, and I think this could delay the process of rigorous scientific inquiry. The urgency of this whole problem is quite overwhelming and is one of the reasons we want to rush the research process. Whatever we can do to develop some sort of effective therapy is of tremendous importance toward realizing the whole goal. The scientific method—the process—however, is essential. That process has worked and needs to be constantly modified and discussed, but it is an open process. People should comment on study designs and have Institutional Review Boards (IRBs) scrutinizing the methods and study design, all to the patient's benefit. If everyone can be involved in the process, the potential for making an error can be reduced.

Question

What are the physicians' and researchers' responsibility to the research subject with AIDS, what is the significance of the research protocol to the individual, and to what extent is informed consent required? For example, a man I spoke with in San Francisco is in the suramin drug study; his physicians told him, "No problem, you won't have any problems continuing your career while you are enrolled in the study." As this man was, other people are severely disabled by suramin. Also, in the interferon trials, there are many complications from treatment with interferon.

Answer

Every IRB and clinical investigator should address these issues. We try to do so in our interferon studies. Our informed consent form has been through our own IRB and through others as well; we point out the side effects of interferon. We never ask a potential participant to sign the informed consent on his first visit. We ask the patient to go home, read the informed consent, talk about it with whomever he wants (including us); we then attempt to address any questions he may have. After these discussions, the patient has to make a decision about whether to participate. Some side effects of drugs are not anticipated in advance. We include all the known side effects that we are aware of in the informed consent.

It is quite common for research subjects not to recall the details of the informed consent interaction. Like other human beings, they have selective memories and remember what they want to remember. Part of the federal regulations that govern clinical trials require the subject to be given a copy of the consent form. It might be worthwhile asking for that form, and reviewing it with the subject. If there are substantive omissions, then an error has been made. You should probably then call the participant and say, "I think we left something out." This type of miscommunication has happened too often to believe that it is all on the hearing side; I am certain it is still a problem, even with a carefully drafted document on informed consent.

Question

I sense that many of the leading hospice programs in this country are not providing effective palliative terminal care for AIDS patients. Many of the pain and symptom management issues are not being adequately provided for.

Answer

The psychosocial aspects of the disease, including depression and anxiety, have not been addressed in their full implications. Even in the research setting, many of the human support aspects of care are not adequately provided for or thought about. That is a justifiable criticism. Good research and good care should go hand in hand.

One has to be constantly reminded that other aspects of this disease become apparent in these studies—depression, anxiety, side effects of medications, etc. The studies, on occasion, are interrupted if the side effects are too overwhelming. Also, a compelling reason explaining why people participate in AIDS studies is that even though a treatment does not turn out to be a good one, it may help to dispel the feeling of being a helpless victim. The people are trying to help themselves and others through their participation in the studies, even though they realize the risks and benefits of participating. In turn, we attempt to build a constructive atmosphere about being involved in the study and to maintain the support that creates this good natured and constructive feeling. Many good things from a broad team approach are helping to address the entire patient, not only the medical aspects.

Question

What role will the research establishment play in guaranteeing, through systems other than just their particular research protocols, the rights and safety of the people who participate in these projects? Some groups at risk have been abused in the past as research subjects, not by an individual per se, but by the whole system in the manner in which they help to develop the data and participate in making a vaccine, yet do not get the direct benefits of the therapy. What should the role of researchers be in developing public policy and teaching the population at large about the value of the population that is generating this information, such that a cure for this illness is found? What are your responsibilities as researchers to take the larger view and say, "We want Congress to do something about guaranteeing the civil rights of these people who are going to be providing the information we so desperately need."

Answer

One of the justifications for performing research on "vulnerable" populations is that those who bear the burdens of research should be the first in line to receive the benefits. This is most commonly said at the "policy" levels, by ethical code or development groups, or in recommendations by national commissions. In fact, in the polio vaccine trial, there was the commitment made that the children who received placebos—if the vaccine proved safe and effective—would be the first to get the polio vaccine should it remain in limited supply. In general, in the sort of research being done today, those who are eligible to be research subjects are those who are most likely to need the benefits that arise out of the research. People who are not in the at-risk populations, in general, will not be competing for interferon-alpha, should it prove to work.

With regard to whether individual researchers can appeal to Congress to reduce the vulnerabilities of these populations, I do not know if they can do this effectively. Some people involved in research have taken it upon themselves to lobby for these issues. The vast majority of researchers are not particularly skilled or knowledgeable about lobbying. Most researchers do what they can to minimize discrimination within their own research environment. I am not certain they can do a lot more. A law may be changed, but that has very little to do with attitudes and prejudice. I would hope that by virtue of performing quality research that demonstrates the diversity and strengths of the subject population, a beneficial effect for the people who are participating would be produced. The quality of the science, at this juncture, is the most critical aspect of the scientist's task.

Protection of Personal Rights

Jeffrey Levi
National Gay Task Force

I believe that, if properly handled, the rights of the individual and the rights of society need not come into conflict. Indeed, proper public health policy will take into account the needs of its individual members. The advent of AIDS has had a profound impact on concepts of public health, for the medical community, for research subjects, and especially for relationships between gay individuals. Because AIDS is affecting the homosexual population so dramatically, and because historically this group does not have a "respected" position in society, the gay population tends to look at the medical community differently from the traditional heterosexual patient or research subject. Whether it is the practicing physician or the public health commissioner, the gay community does not imbue medical science with the same total faith and trust that the medical community typically tends to receive. The medical community has not always been their friend. Not much more than 10 years ago, for example, the American Psychiatric Association classified homosexuality as a mental disorder. The same U.S. Public Health Service that is now working with varying degrees of energy and effectiveness on AIDS, that is asking us to trust them with these issues and rely on their expertise, is the same U.S. Public Health Service that continues to enforce the ban against entry of homosexuals into the United States. This ban is based, incidentally, on the claim that homosexuals are psychopathic personalities. This sort of attitudinal perspective, especially when addressing issues of confidentiality, is relevant when attempting to establish relationships between individuals and the health care community. To make progress in the science of this disease, we must make the research more sensitive and bring about a much higher degree of cooperation between the research subject and the researcher. If the researcher is armed with a better understanding of the gay population in society, then I believe that research will be more productive and the end results will be better.

Let me share with you the basis for some of those concerns. We often call this our "Homo 101" course; invariably, it bears repeating again and again. Simply being identified as homosexual in the United States leaves one vulnerable to discrimination and rejection. AIDS researchers are asking for even more. They ask for information about our lifestyles and activities that could result not only in discrimination but criminal prosecution as well. The courts have consistently ruled that lesbians and gay men do not have the same rights to equal protection under the law that other Americans enjoy. Private employers have the right to discharge employees simply because they are gay or lesbian, unless there are local laws banning discrimination based on sexual orientation. The federal government itself discriminates against gay people, despite the fact that federally funded researchers are asking their subjects to reveal highly privileged and personal information about their homosexuality. Gays and lesbians are automatically discharged from the military. Many federal agencies deny security clearances to people who are gay, even if they are openly gay and are not susceptible to blackmail. When we discuss a sexually transmitted disease such as AIDS, we are entering another area where the legal status of homosexuals makes us even more vulnerable. Consensual homosexual activity is still illegal, usually a felony, in 23 states and in the District of Columbia. Sharing information with researchers about sexual activity may be vital to learning about AIDS, but the willingness of the research subject to share that information will be directly related to assurances on the part of the researcher that this information will not be shared with local prosecutors.

The vulnerability of gay people is intensified by the AIDS crisis. Irrational fears about AIDS have led to blanket discrimination against gay men. The mere identification with someone who has AIDS has resulted in job discrimination, loss of a household, and other blatant forms of discrimination. It is ironic, however, that people with AIDS seem to have more legal protection than gay people do generally. People with AIDS are considered to be disabled, and are therefore protected by laws against discrimination of the disabled. If you are gay, or in some other way identified with a person with AIDS, but actually do not have the disease, you may not have the same legal recourse available.

Perhaps, by way of example, the serious and very real nature of AIDS discrimination may be emphasized. A man in the Navy, stationed in Puerto Rico, was identified as having AIDS. His physician said to him, "Tell me, are you gay? You can trust me." The Navy man said, "Yes, I am gay," and proceeded to list three sexual contacts within the Navy. What this patient did not know is that in the military, there is no doctrine of physician–patient confidentiality. The physician promptly turned the information over to naval intelligence. This person was transferred to Bethesda where he is allegedly getting hospital care, but at the same time he is being required to discuss all that he knows about homosexuality in the Navy. He has been told by the Navy that "We will not prosecute you. We will not single you out. We will not give you a dishonorable discharge and therefore take away all of your potential medical benefits," which he obviously needs desperately now that he has AIDS. "However, you must identify all the other people in the military whom you know to be gay." The use of the screening blood test opens up a wide spectrum of dangerous and potentially damaging approaches to discriminate further against people solely on the basis of their sexual orientation.

In New York City, the board of directors of a cooperative building attempted to evict a well-respected physician who performed research on AIDS from his medical office, claiming that patients walking through the building lobby lowered property values and endangered tenants by exposing them to AIDS. This matter was settled successfully. In Washington, D.C., an openly gay man with a history of sexual transmitted disease has been denied life insurance coverage because the life insurance company claims the man is at risk for AIDS. In Arkansas, a lesbian mother is fighting to keep custody of her children. The father of the children has raised the argument that to allow them to remain with their mother threatens them with exposure to AIDS. These examples, while seemingly irrational and unreasonable, are useful to orient people to the context in which we are working.

Ever increasing demands from the gay community for greater protections of confidentiality are being made. The Centers for Disease Control (CDC) performs a surveillance function collecting data on contagious diseases for use in developing public health policy aimed at addressing these trends. After fairly extensive negotiations with the CDC, we were successful in receiving an assurance of confidentiality from CDC that protects from a subpoena any of the information that is shared as part of the surveillance process. This is a sensible approach, especially when one considers that surveillance data are collected for public health reasons rather than to support prosecution of the victim. Many physicians would be unwilling to share or report as accurately as one might want or need for surveillance purposes without that kind of assurance. Many patients are going to be quite unwilling to share that kind of information without similar sorts of confidentiality protections. Unfortunately, this type of protection has not been extended to federally funded research, and the assurance of confidentiality is for surveillance purposes only.

Some types of federal research receive a certificate of confidentiality which gives the researcher the right not to reveal information requested in a subpoena; however, the individual researcher makes the decision whether to comply with the subpoena or not. In light of the risks that medical information will be made available pursuant to a subpoena, it is imperative that the participant be fully informed in advance of the risks of participating in a given research study. Researchers must make clear to the potential research subjects the risks of private medical information being revealed if the researcher receives a subpoena. If a researcher has a certificate of confidentiality, or an assurance that allows the withholding of documents relating to AIDS research, then the research subject should have the researcher sign a contract, through the use of the informed consent form, to compel the investigator not to share privileged information. If the certificates of confidentiality or other legal protections against sharing information are not in place, then the participant should be fully informed of the full extent of the risks of revealing information. The research subject should be informed that pursuant to a court order, the information might have to be shared.

Another approach to preventing the release of highly sensitive, confidential information is through the legislative process. We are working now with several legislators in Washington, D.C., to develop legislation to protect the confidential information released in research on AIDS. At the moment, the primary stumbling block is that the Public Health Service is not supporting the development of protections of the medical information for AIDS subjects. We hope that dispute will be resolved in time.

It has been very difficult to heighten public awareness to some of these fears. The stigma we experience as gay people and as people in a high risk group to contract AIDS, are a major part of it. In a peculiar sort of way, the development of the HTLV-III antibody test has altered the public perception of the confidentiality issue through discussions in the straight press. The most likely explanation for this group's attention must stem from the possibility that some non-gay, non-IV drug users may be falsely classified as HTLV-III positive, due to inaccuracies in the test. The people then begin to understand what the stigmatization is all about.

There might also be greater understanding of our concerns about the test if it were used for the average person, beyond the blood donation process. We know that this blood test is valuable in identifying, sometimes, that a person tested is exposed or infected by the HTLV-III virus. What medical intervention is there? To date, no intervention is useful. Is a recommendation to follow safe sex practices useful? If a person is in a high risk group, they should be following safe sexual practices irrespective of the antibody test result. On the other hand, a negative test result does not necessarily mean that a person has not been infected with the HTLV-III virus—a person may not have seroconverted yet. Anyone who falls into a high risk group should carry on his life as though he were positive without a test result. From the public health standpoint, therefore, there may be less reason for high risk people to be tested. However, people at lesser risk do not know whether they should be following these precautionary sexual practices. Perhaps the true utility of this blood test lies in the health setting—screening people at low risk for AIDS—the purpose of which is to give advice to straight people about safe sex practices. It is very easy to tell gay people to adopt safe sex practices and to use condoms. Is the White House and the Department of Health and Human Services going to tell straight people to visit Planned Parenthood and find out how to use a condom? While this is a facetious suggestion, it usually encourages people to consider the gay person's perspective and assists people in gaining a clearer sense of the societal and psychosocial implications of this blood test, and of AIDS.

Lastly, when we talk about changes in behavior because of HTLV-III antibody positivity, we cannot tell people to give up sex or sexual expression. We are telling people that they have to change the way they express themselves sexually. Safe sex is now a medical necessity, and it is here to stay. Initially, because the message was coming from straight, primarily government scientists, it was dismissed as homophobia. Unfortunately, it is an accurate description of a deadly disease that touches very private notions of sexuality, and it is very hard for people to understand and accept. The notion of safe and more restrictive sex is easier if you believe that all people, gay and non-gay alike, are going to have to adapt their sexual practices and expression. Because of AIDS, there is going to be a second kind of sexual revolution in this country—one that is clearly more restrictive and much more difficult to accept.

Ethical and Moral Issues in AIDS Research

Jerome E. Groopman, M.D.
Assistant Professor of Medicine
Harvard Medical School
Member, Mayor's and State Task Force on AIDS

AIDS research does not involve an abstract process or activity divorced from the reality that confronts AIDS victims. There is a tremendous amount of respect, and, indeed, bravery, among those individuals who participate in AIDS research. For the AIDS victim, the individual benefits from participating in a clinical trial are often difficult to ascertain. Similarly, noninfected individuals serving as "controls," or others who serve as controls because they test serum positive for the virus yet do not have symptoms of the illness, give generously of their time. Many of these people have already gone through the psychological process of confronting their illness and are very motivated to engage in research for personal reasons.

One of the difficulties in coping with AIDS research relates to the benefits it may provide. We have been attempting to understand the biology of the virus and the biology of cofactors that interact with the virus, in an effort to modulate the clinical outcome after infection. Through further research we may be able to understand why some individuals who are exposed become quite ill, while others carry the virus yet do not seem to suffer any adverse consequences. Apparently, there are different levels of susceptibility or incubation periods that we do not understand. Antibody positivity may mean that within a given person, there are dormant viral sequences that have not yet been expressed. Perhaps some individuals are more susceptible to the virus; perhaps a given strain of virus is more virulent or more efficiently transmitted to others than a different strain. These problems are obviously very important questions for the individual and for society. The only way to derive answers to these problems is to perform careful research.

Many of the individuals involved in AIDS research appear to feel a tremendous responsibility to AIDS victims, their friends, families, and sexual contacts. Part of this feeling of duty to the patient stems from a concern about the tremendous psychological stress they must learn to cope with. Four years ago, I was transfused during an operation in California. I had no sexual risk, but always lurking in the minds of all health care providers is the thought that, despite the negative studies and the reassuring data from the Centers for Disease Control, could you be the first health care worker to contract the disease? I was more concerned about the possibility of transmitting the virus through the transfusion than I was concerned about exposure to the disease as a health care provider. Nevertheless, I became concerned about the safety of my wife and my son. In retrospect, this concern was somewhat irrational; it was also highly stressful. I tested HTLV-III negative, and was tremendously relieved. The experience made me highly sensitive to the kinds of stresses that must exist in the homosexual community and, I think, in the heterosexual community as well.

Since we feel we need to perform research in order to prevent future diseases, what are we able to do for people in light of the current state of knowledge? Clearly, as the science progresses, the issues will change. With our present knowledge base, I believe that we have certain obligations. First, we are obligated to continue researching relevant issues. Next, we must develop safeguards for patient rights of confidentiality. Within the institutions performing research, there must be careful considerations about protecting the confidentiality of the research participants. Special legislation should be considered. This is an unusual, deadly epidemic which poses unique questions. It may be a mistake to rely on legal responses derived in response to earlier available medical precedents, such as cholera epidemics, leprosy, or syphilis. Perhaps patience, understanding, and careful research may benefit the victims; legislative assistance in protecting their rights would be a useful supplement.

The Effects of Discrimination Against Gays

Michael Callen
Co-Founder, Gay Men with AIDS
Founding Member, People with AIDS
Member, New York States AIDS Advisory Council

There continues to be considerable confusion about the relationship between HTLV-III antibody positivity and the disease of AIDS. Why do some people with antibodies to the virus become ill while others do not? Many of the social ill effects and the complicated issues which have arisen have occurred because of the erroneous public perception that if a person is HTLV-III positive, then the person has or can transmit AIDS. What appears to be potentially transmissible is the HTLV-III virus. Whether or not an infected person develops AIDS probably depends on other, confounding, and as yet unknown cofactors.

Another important consideration that appears to be overlooked, or at least underrated, by AIDS researchers, is the importance of the social context in which the disease and the research is occurring. The country is riding a wave of conservatism. The population affected by AIDS is being studied by researchers whose money is coming from the federal government. I suggest that a lot of what we know about this disease is based on epidemiology that may be suspect for a number of reasons. How likely is it that a person interviewed by a federal researcher will admit truthfully to illegal sexual acts, illicit drug use, or acts of prostitution? Researchers often naively assume that people with AIDS and their controls have told the truth. This bias may be profound and persuasive enough to invalidate a considerable amount of the data that are being gathered.

Another area where researchers and public health officials are being led astray is in the area of heterosexual transmission of AIDS by prostitutes. As an example, the health commissioner from New York City has emphatically and repeatedly stated that he does not know of a single case of AIDS in the city of New York where the sole risk factor is having used the services of a prostitute. Can you imagine a prostitute cooperating with a federal or government researcher? The very idea is as ludicrous as a homosexual in the Navy admitting to Navy personnel that he is gay. It simply is not done. We must think in terms of seriously questioning the quality of the data because of the social context in which AIDS research is occurring.

Further, it is easy to underrate the profound effects that the study and treatment of people with AIDS has on the treating and research physicians and other health care professionals. The last time I was in the hospital—I am part of one of the long research projects being conducted in New York—one of the physicians who is performing research in this area spoke to me as a friend, rather than as a researcher. He confessed that he had not had sex in over two years, and that he had realized, in talking to me, that the reason that he was avoiding sex was because he was afraid that he might be HTLV-III positive. Although he had access to the test, he had not tested himself. His somewhat irrational feeling that he might be HTLV-III positive was having a profoundly negative effect on his ability to interact socially. This example reflects another aspect of how this disease is adversely affecting so many peoples' lives.

Comment

I am Pastoral Care Coordinator for AIDS patients, at the St. Luke's-Roosevelt Hospital in New York City, and am aware that at the St. Luke's site of our hospital, and at a growing number of New York City hospitals, one-third to one-half of our AIDS patients come, not from the gay community, but primarily from the IV drug abuse population. Whereas the gay community knows about "safe sex," IV drug abusers know about neither safe sex nor safe needles. I think there are myriad educational, ethical, and public health issues relating to the drug subculture that we have not even begun to address. I hope we do not focus solely on the risk to the gay people, because I believe that it is much more in the drug community that we have only begun to see the tip of the iceberg. What is being done in San Francisco is terrific. However, in New York, the drug cofactor is a powerfully hard one to get a handle on, making the New York situation many times more difficult. The CDC is not helping much either, especially when you evaluate the manner in which the AIDS statistics are tabulated. If an AIDS victim is both gay and an IV drug user, he is classified as gay. The CDC statistics do not reflect the significant percentage of those men with AIDS who are gay and also IV drug users.

The government has the same difficulties in overcoming its reluctance to give the safe sex advice to gay men as it does educating IV drug users about the proper use and administration of IV drugs. For example, in Washington, D.C., there were a series of drug overdoses. Apparently, the overdoses were not caused by a contaminated batch of drugs, but by people mixing drugs with alcohol. The police reacted by saying, "Stop shooting up." They could not condone the illegal activity of abusing IV drugs, even though drinking was legal. One of the much simpler things to tell a IV drug user was, "Do not drink if you are going to shoot up." I think we will encounter the same rigid thinking by the government when they realize a serious problem exists when addicts share needles and are transmitting the virus to other addicts. How does a government that will not condone IV drug abuse educate addicts by telling them to use a clean needle?

It is extraordinarily difficult to achieve behavior modification in a community such as the IV drug abusers. In the gay community, there is clearly a very high level of awareness, education, and organization. That does not exist in the intravenous drug community. It is probably even more incumbent upon the health authorities, however, to organize strong educational programs in the high schools, and in many areas of New York City, about the dangers of drug abuse, which now obviously have expanded to include the acquisition of the virus.

Question

In the confidentiality realm, we spoke very briefly to the issue of voluntary violation of confidentiality by the researchers. I have had the personal experience of attending two recent meetings dealing with ethical aspects of AIDS, one at the Hastings Center and one meeting arranged by the National Institutes of Health, in New York, for Institutional Review Board participants, with four distinguished medical scientists participating. One of them was the director of a federal laboratory who said that if any subject of research revealed that he or she had committed a crime, they would report that person directly to the authorities. I know that 95% of the people who are answering our research questions have, by definition, committed a felony in many states by either possessing or using illicit substances or committing homosexual acts. When I asked whether they would tell their subjects that they intended to report them to the authorities if they revealed the truth, they said of course not, that this would spoil the study. These investigators seemed horrendously insensitive, which only seems to compound the fear of the participants.

Answer

(Sheldon Landesman, M.D.): I think the issue is certainly a valid one, although I would suggest that it is probably no different with research on AIDS than it is with any other form of research.

A comment was made about viewing blood donation as more an issue of trust and not as a contract, and I think to some extent, no matter how you describe it, the relationship between a researcher and a research participant is also something that is based upon trust. The research participant is donating knowledge about himself, private information, or his blood in a manner similar to a blood donor, and ultimately if there isn't a certain element of trust in there, none of this research could proceed. There will always be researchers who will violate that trust. Perhaps one of the salutory outcomes of this epidemic is to enhance the researcher's sensitivity to this aspect of their ethical obligations. Our primary obligation to our research subjects is to protect them. They have volunteered to donate blood and give us information for their own benefit and ultimately for the benefit of society. I feel under no obligation to anyone to breach their confidences.

A serious question could arise if a person in a research study who has AIDS might be acting irresponsibly and donating blood for money. If you have a research subject who you know is HTLV-III virus positive and, therefore, theoretically can communicate the disease or the virus to other persons, I do not think you can prevent him from engaging in certain sexual activities. I think your job as a researcher, if you have established a good relationship, is to educate him as much as you possibly can as to his social responsibilities. In the overwhelming number of cases, this effort will probably suffice. I like to believe that people on a one-to-one basis are oftentimes very socially responsible.

Confidentiality and AIDS Research
Where Research and Personal Rights Conflict

Carol Levine, M.A.
Editor, *The Hastings Center Report*
Managing Editor, *IRB: A Review of Human Subjects Research*
Chair, AIDS Medical Foundation Investigational Review Board

A problem that has been stated many times yet bears further discussion relates to the conflict between the needs of researchers, who hope to benefit society, and the rights of individuals who want to protect their privacy. This conflict in the AIDS area became very apparent to us at the Hastings Center a few years ago when we began receiving concerned calls from both researchers and potential research subjects who expressed serious questions about the extent to which confidentiality could be guaranteed. We tried to answer these inquiries on an ad hoc basis, but we quickly concluded that more systemic issues were being raised and that we had to try to deal with them in a systematic way. We were fortunate enough to receive a funding grant from the Charles A. Dana Foundation to prepare a series of guidelines on confidentiality and AIDS research, which are included here in the appendix to this part.

We began by meeting with a group of consultants in an effort to define the scope and perception of the problem. A much larger group, including researchers, public health officials, physicians treating AIDS patients, representatives of at-risk groups, ethicists, lawyers, social scientists, and some members of the blood banking community were asked to participate. We solicited comments about the various perspectives on confidentiality. A discussion draft was prepared and discussed at a meeting of these experts.

On some of the points, there was a clear consensus. Recommendation 7, for example, under the heading "Who Should Not Have Access to Personally Identifiable Information Obtained in Researcher Surveillance" reflected the group consensus.

> No individual, organization or agency should have access to any personally identifiable information gathered in research or surveillance on AIDS for any purpose other than AIDS research or surveillance without the consent of the individuals or the subjects.

We wanted to recommend precluding the release of any information gathered for the specific purpose of AIDS research or surveillance to any other government agency or employers, landlords, and others. The subject populations were very worried about this type of dissemination of research data, because it could harm them. The commentators agreed that the recommendation was appropriate and necessary.

In general, the guidelines state that every institution conducting research should have a clearly stated and enforced policy addressing the security of records, how identifiers will be handled, and the eventual disposition of the medical records. We recommended that researchers resist subpoenas that seek the compulsory disclosure of identifiable information. We added that while current safeguards are inadequate and will require legislative and regulatory change, they do provide researchers with some grounds for resisting efforts to force the disclosure of research records with personally identifiable information. We felt that courts would be likely to review such efforts to resist subpoenas more favorably if the researcher had established that confidentiality was an important part of the research itself. In order to protect fully the confidentiality of research subjects in AIDS studies, administrative and statutory safeguards should be created at federal and state levels to prevent both unjustifiable voluntary and involuntary disclosure of personally identifiable data. In general, the commentators felt it was inadequate to rely on the professional discretion of those safeguarding the records and that legislative protection for the participants was necessary.

On a number of issues, irrespective of the various ways in which we approached the area of concern, we were unable to develop a consensus. For example, we recommended that individual researchers select the type of patient/participant identifiers, if necessary, that provide maximum protection of confidentiality. We could not reach a consensus on the use of Social Security numbers as these identifiers. The Social Security number offers the greatest potential for matching data sets; it also seems to pose the greatest threat to confidentiality. Those who supported the use of Social Security numbers pointed out that these identifiers are more specific than names. For that reason alone, some researchers believe that Social Security numbers are indispensable in longitudinal studies. But those who opposed the use of Social Security numbers stressed that those numbers are assigned and held by the federal government and that potential misuse of the information is a very serious fear. In light of this fear, we also could not agree as to whether private agencies or federal agencies are the best place to hold the identifiers.

Another question about which we could not reach a consensus was whether Investigational Review Boards (IRBs) or the investigators should be responsible for considering the concerns about risks of the subject populations. According to federal law, IRBs are required to review the protocols in an effort to minimize the risk of harm to the study participant. In this respect, the IRBs are responsible. The discussants could not agree, however, about the scope of the IRB's duty. The dispute centered on whether the IRB members themselves should interview representatives of the subject populations or whether they should only ascertain that the investigators have done so. This dispute created a very serious division in the group; we concluded that someone should conduct the interviews and that the IRB has the responsibility to insure that the interviews are done. We did not decide whether the interviews should be performed by the IRB or not.

One underlying issue that we did resolve is whether AIDS is a special situation that requires special constraints on researchers. I believe that special constraints and interviews with subjects, among other things, are more important in this type of research. However, I think an additional by-product of our work was the recognition that all research data need stronger confidentiality protections and that the specific problems raised in the AIDS area are representative of problems in medical research generally.

References

1. Paul, J.R. 1971. *A history of polio-myelitis*. New Haven: Yale University Press.
2. Boston Interhospital Virus Study Group and NIAID Sponsored Cooperative Antiviral Clinical Study. 1975. Failure of high dose 5-iodo-2'-deoxyuridine (IDU) in the therapy of herpes simplex virus encephalitis: evidence of unacceptable toxicity. *New England Journal of Medicine* 292:599–603.
3. Hirsch, M.S., and R.T. Schooley. 1983. Treatment of herpesvirus infections. *New England Journal of Medicine* 309:963–970, 1034–1039.
4. Peabody, Francis. 1927. The care of the patient. The Gay lecture on medical ethics. Quoted by George Packer Berry in, Remarks on the reopening of the Thorndike Memorial Laboratory. An unpublished lecture, Harvard Medical School, 1964.
5. Szmuness, Wolf, Cladd E. Stevens, Edward J. Harley, et al. 1980. Hepatitis B vaccine: Demonstration of efficacy in a controlled clinical trial in a high risk population in the United States. *New England Journal of Medicine* 303:833–841.
6. Rudstein, David. 1970. The ethical design of human experiments. In *Experimentation with human subjects,* ed. Paul A. Freund. New York: George Braziller.

Appendix
Guidelines for Confidentiality
in Research on AIDS

Ronald Bayer, Carol Levine, and Thomas H. Murray*

The identification of Acquired Immune Deficiency Syndrome (AIDS) three years ago created a crisis of confidence. Persons with AIDS and others who might be research subjects recognize that research is essential to understand, treat, and prevent this devastating disease; yet they are concerned that information disclosed for research purposes might be used in ways detrimental to their interests. Unless they have confidence in the systems designed to protect their privacy and in the people to whom personal information is entrusted, they will face a difficult choice: either to provide inaccurate or incomplete data, thus compromising the validity of the research; or to give accurate and full data, thus placing themselves at risk. The problem, then, is: What procedures and policies will both protect the privacy of research subjects and enable research to proceed expeditiously? Now that major research efforts are being undertaken to tackle the many puzzling aspects of AIDS, this question has become an urgent one, and these guidelines are designed to address it.

While in part a technical and administrative problem, the issue has important ethical, legal, and social aspects as well. Ethically, a balance must be struck between the principle of respect for persons (which requires that individuals should be treated as autonomous agents who have the right to control their own destinies), and the pursuit of the common good (which requires maximizing possible benefits and minimizing possible harms, to society as well as to individuals). Legally—by statute, policy, and regulation—subjects, researchers, and institutions must be protected from involuntary disclosure of information. Those entrusted with confidential information must be prohibited by law from unjustifiable voluntary disclosure. As a society we must express our moral commitment to the principle that all persons are due a full measure of compassion and respect.

Any investigation involving a possibly communicable disease poses a tension between an individual's desire to control personal information and the desire of others to have access to that information. Although this tension is not unique to AIDS, it is particularly sharply drawn in this case because those groups that have been identified as at high risk are also highly vulnerable socially, economically, and politically. Because of the unknown factors that are involved in AIDS, researchers may have to explore many intimate aspects of an individual's medi-

---

*Reprinted with permission from *IRB: A Review of Human Subjects Research* 6(6):1–7 (November/ December 1984).

cal, social, and behavioral history and will have to keep these data for an extended period.

Investigators may seek information that reveals, for example, that a subject has engaged in homosexual or other sexual practices that are illegal in many states and are subject to social stigma; has injected drugs obtained illegally; has engaged in criminal activities, such as prostitution; or has entered the country illegally.

Furthermore, disclosure of a diagnosis of AIDS—or perhaps even involvement in AIDS research—carries a stigma that can adversely affect a person's interests socially, politically, and economically. Potential subjects, either individually or through organizations representing their interests, have sought recognition of these risks and assurances that appropriate measures will be taken to protect their privacy.

For these reasons we believe that special guidelines are necessary for AIDS research. These guidelines are concerned with the protection of the privacy of persons with AIDS and their families and friends, with the confidentiality of information collected about them, and with the security of data systems in which this information is stored. However, research into other diseases also carries risks for subject populations. We hope that these guidelines will stimulate an examination of the general problem of protecting confidentiality of research records.

AIDS research will be conducted in a context of standards already set by law and regulation, professional practice, and agency policy. In some cases these standards provide only minimal protection. These guidelines, which were developed by a multidisciplinary group representing diverse professional, public and social interests, are intended to strengthen existing protections and procedures. They are directed at several audiences: researchers, public health officials, legislators, members of Institutional Review Boards, subjects, and organizations that represent subjects' interests.

I. What Activities Are Covered by These Guidelines?

These guidelines deal with confidentiality in research on AIDS, which can be distinguished from medical care, surveillance, and public health interventions. *Research* is an activity designed to discover generalizable knowledge. *Medical care* is intended to improve the health and well-being of a patient. *Surveillance* involves systematic collection of data for the purpose of monitoring the incidence and prevalence of a disease. *Public health intervention* are actions taken to halt its spread.

These activities are often intimately related. A patient undergoing medical care may at the same time be a research subject in a study designed to evaluate that care. Designing effective public health interventions depends on the success of research and surveillance. Sometimes information gained in surveillance may be useful in research, while research may identify categories of information that are relevant to surveillance. To complicate matters further, the same government organization—a state or local public health department—is responsible for both surveillance and public health interventions, and for that matter, may be involved in research.

Precisely because of the institutional overlap among research, surveillance, and public health interventions, we feel it is essential to distinguish them from each other, and to state clearly the ethical problems each raises. In research, the two central ethical problems are confidentiality and consent. To the extent that surveillance activities are limited to the collection and interpretation of information about individuals, surveillance resembles (and may be indistinguishable from) research, and the central moral issues are, again, confidentiality and consent. Surveillance, however, may become intimately intertwined with the possibility of public health interventions. The values served by public health intervention— the prevention of harm and the promotion of the general welfare—can and sometimes do result in compromising confidentiality and consent. Surveillance, then, occupies a problematic middle position between research on the one side and public health interventions on the other.

The ethical issues in public health interventions are beyond the scope of these guidelines. Our concern here is with research and, secondarily, with surveillance. One difficult problem is what to do when information about identifiable individuals gained through research or surveillance might be sought for public health interventions. We address this issue in Section VI of these guidelines.

II. For Whom Is Confidentiality Protection Necessary?

These guidelines should be applied to all individuals, regardless of citizenship status, who become the subjects of AIDS-related research or surveillance. This includes:

1. all individuals meeting the Centers for Disease Control's definition of AIDS—that is, who have the disease in a clearly recognizable form;

2. all individuals suspected of having, developing, or being at risk for AIDS, for example those with lymphadenopathy, reversed T-cell ratios or other suggestive evidence of AIDS;

3. all people involved in research studies as controls;

4. all persons interviewed or otherwise contacted in the course of AIDS-related research or surveillance, for whatever reason.

III. What Kinds of Information Are Researchers Likely to Need and What Are the Likely Sources?

Information relevant to AIDS research may be of many kinds and may come from numerous sources. Researchers may need, for example, information about an individual's medical condition, medical history, sexual practices, country of origin, and drug use. Such information may be obtained from, for example, interviews with patients, friends, and relatives; physicians' records; hospital records; administrative records (for example, insurance claims); records gathered by other researchers; and records gathered by public health agencies.

IV. When Are Identifiers Needed in Research and What Precautions Should Be Taken?

"Identifiers" are coded or uncoded pieces of information that enable a researcher to recognize that different sets of data have come from the same individual. Some kinds of identifiers—names or Social Security numbers, for example—can be directly linked to specific individuals. A second type employs technical devices—for example, encoding names, deleting some important part of an individual's name, or relying on subject-created aliases—for making the identification of a specific individual difficult or nearly impossible, while still permitting sets of data to be matched.

The need for identifiers may create a conflict with individuals' interests in protecting their privacy. This conflict can be minimized in several ways:

Recommendation 1: **Researchers should determine whether identifiers are essential to carry out their research.**

Identifiers are not necessary in all research. For example, a study that involves only a single interview or a single compilation of statistical data may not need identifiers. Identifiers are necessary when: (a) the researcher may need to inform a research subject about a medical condition requiring treatment; (b) the researcher requires linking one set of data with other sets; (c) the researcher requires linking information gathered at different times; or (d) the researcher requires verifying the reliability of the data.

When the decision is made to keep identifiers, the question as to who shall hold them—government or private institutions—remains controversial. It is not clear which party would be better able to protect confidentiality, and this matter deserves further discussion.

Recommendation 2: **Researchers should select the form of identifier that provides maximum protection of individuals' identities commensurate with responsible research.**

Among the characteristics of identifiers that researchers should consider is the feasibility of deductive disclosure—the possibility of deducing the identity of a particular individual from the combination of a coded identifier and other information. We know of no scheme that provides complete immunity from the possibility of deductive disclosure. However, careful attention to limiting the information given out in connection with coded identifiers can make deductive disclosure so technically difficult, or so cumbersome and costly, as to make it practically unfeasible.

The group that considered these guidelines did not reach a consensus on the use of Social Security numbers in AIDS research. Social Security numbers offer the greatest potential for matching data sets; they also pose the greatest threat to confidentiality. Those who supported the use of Social Security numbers pointed out that these identifiers are more specific than names. For that reason some researchers believe that Social Security numbers are indispensable in longitudinal studies, where it is important to be able to recognize that different sets of data have come from a single person. Those who oppose the use of Social Security numbers stress that these numbers are assigned and held by the federal government. Potential misuse of information by government agencies is one of the strongest fears expressed by subjects in AIDS research. This issue needs further exploration, and we suggest that the continuing advisory board recommended to examine ethical issues in AIDS research address it. (See Section XII.)

Recommendation 3: **Researchers should explain to research participants why identifiers are needed in a given instance, what system of confidentiality protection is in place, and how it works.**

Recommendation 4: **When coded identifiers are to be used, research records should be stripped of personal identifiers as soon as the information is received.**

In studies in which coding has been determined to be necessary, subjects are at risk as long as personally identified material is retained in the record.

V. Who Should Have Access to Personally Identifiable Information Obtained in Research or Surveillance?

Recommendation 5: **Only those engaged in AIDS-related research or surveillance should have access to personally identifiable information.**

Even those with such legitimate purposes will not always need the information in a form where the individual's identity is not disguised or deleted. (See Section IV on Identifiers.)

Recommendation 6: **Research data in personally identifiable form should be redisclosed to investigators in another research project only (a) with the informed consent of the subject or a person authorized to give permission on** the subject's behalf, and (b) after it has been ascertained that the additional research project protects confidentiality at least as well as the original research.

Researchers commonly share data without identifiers; this practice permits research information to be useful to others involved in related studies. Consent for disclosure without identifiers is not necessarily required. However, when redisclosure with identifiable data is proposed for additional research, researchers have a responsibility to assure that confidentiality is at least as well protected after redisclosure as it was originally and they should not redisclose the data without consent of the subject or someone designated by the subject. Because of the possibility that many current AIDS subjects may die, IRBs should consider appropriate mechanisms to protect these subjects' privacy interests after death. For example, they may require a proxy to be named by the dying patient to consent to redisclosure of personally identifiable material.

VI. Who Should NOT Have Access to Personally Identifiable Information Obtained in Research or Surveillance.

Recommendation 7: **No individual, organization, or agency should have access to any personally identifiable information gathered in research or surveillance on AIDS for any purpose other than AIDS research or surveillance without the consent of the individuals who are the subjects of the information.**

Under no circumstances should personally identifiable information about the subjects of research or surveillance be given to any individual, organization, or agency where there is a reasonable expectation that the use of the information might be harmful to the interests of the subjects. This would preclude releasing identifiable subject records to the Department of Justice or Defense, the Internal Revenue Service, or the Immigration and Naturalization Service; to local or state law enforcement agencies; or to employers, landlords, or other private individuals or institutions.

There are two possible exceptions to this prohibition on release of personally identifiable records. The first is for the scientific and financial audit of research, which is mandated by law for federally funded research. (See Section VII.)

The second possible exception is for an as yet unforeseen occasion where specific individuals are known to be at preventable risk for the disease, and where information contained in research records is uniquely necessary to protect them. Such an event is unlikely; still, we believe it will usually be possible to protect the identities of research participants through one of a variety of methods.

Because of the growing evidence linking blood transfusions and the transmission of AIDS, the possible contamination of blood and blood products with a hypothetical infectious agent may pose the first such case. Consider this possible scenario: A researcher has obtained detailed information that AIDS patients had donated blood before they were diagnosed, and blood banks and public health officials want access to that information. This request might meet most or all of the conditions mentioned in the preceding paragraph. Research may have confirmed that specific individuals—those who would receive the blood or blood products—are at risk for AIDS; that risk would be prevented by destroying the contaminated blood. Furthermore, the only source of the information might be the research records. Even then disclosure should be guided by the principle of giving the most limited amount of information necessary to accomplish the task of identifying the contaminated blood samples. The researcher could, for example, give the names and perhaps the dates of donation to those centers where the person with AIDS reported having given blood. All other information gained in the research, not pertinent to the immediate problem, should remain confidential. The blood banks in turn should keep confidential the names of donors with AIDS given to them by the researcher.

We have not discussed in detail all the ethical issues related to AIDS and blood donation; this is an issue that needs immediate attention.

VII. What Are the Current Legal Protections?

Researchers and subjects share a concern that data collected in the course of investigations into, and the surveillance of, AIDS will be disclosed involuntarily as a result of subpoena or other legal procedures. These fears have some justification. Although a variety of legislative enactments at federal and state levels have been designed to provide some degree of protection of privacy, the legal status of the confidentiality of research records remains ambiguous in many circumstances.

At the federal level, the Freedom of Information Act (5 U.S.C. 552, 1982) and the Privacy Act of 1974 (5 U.S.C. 552a, 1982) establish rules governing the disclosure of data held by the federal government. These two laws operate together to prohibit the public disclosure of medical information in federal files. There are procedural and substantive safeguards against other uses and disclosures of medical information, but the protections are not as strong as the protections against public disclosure. Agencies have some discretion in deciding on collateral uses of records. Records held by state agencies and private parties are generally not subject to these federal laws.

Stronger protections are available to the subjects of research under other federal regulations. The Centers for Disease Control may under special circumstances issue a confidentiality certificate when it seeks data from researchers in order to guarantee the privacy of the requested records (Section 308 [d] of the

Public Health Service Act, 42 U.S.C. 242 m). Research subjects involved in studies funded by the Alcohol, Drug Abuse and Mental Health Administration may also be afforded greater confidentiality (42 C.F.R. Sec 2.1). Most stringent are the requirements of grants made by the National Institute of Justice, which not only protect researchers from subpoena, but prohibit them from disclosing identifiable research data (42 U.S.C. 3789g).

Some states have sought to protect the confidentiality of research records through legislation. In New York State, for example, the statute that amended the public health laws to create the New York State AIDS Institute (S. 5930, passed June 26, 1983) stipulated that all projects funded by that agency guarantee the confidentiality of data collected on all identifiable individuals.

Such protections against disclosure by researchers are qualified by the legal requirement that records be made available to those governmental entities charged with the responsibility of conducting scientific and financial audits or program evaluations. Under current regulations, for example, the Food and Drug Administration may examine the records of clinical investigations being conducted under New Drug Applications (21 U.S.C. 374 [a], sec. 704[a]), and the Inspector General of the Department of Health and Human Services may examine the research records of most federally funded research projects (42 U.S.C. 3525).

The creation of publicly held records on persons with AIDS as a result of surveillance conducted by local and state health departments raises special problems. With AIDS a reportable disease in over thirty states, public health officials have attempted to protect their records from the scrutiny of governmental agencies that might want to learn the names of those who have been reported by physicians and hospitals. In New York City, for example, the Board of Health created protections against unwarranted disclosure by amending the New York City Health Code (Sec. 11.07, subsec. [a] and [b]) on August 25, 1983, extending to AIDS the same safeguards already in place for reports of venereal diseases, narcotics addiction and drug abuse. Such records "are not subject to subpoena or to inspection by persons other than authorized personnel of the [Health] Department."

The strength of state and local protections, however, is unknown, since they have not been challenged in court by federal authorities.

VIII: What Steps Should Be Taken to Enhance the Legal Protections Available to Research Subjects?

Recommendation 8: **Researchers, institutions, and IRBs should investigate prevailing statutes and administrative procedures for the protection of the confidentiality of research records in their jurisdictions.**

Given the current level of amibiguity regarding how well local, state, and federal regulations and statutes do in fact protect the confidentiality of research records, a systematic review of such provisions is necessary to evaluate proposed research protocols.

Recommendation 9: **Every institution or agency that conducts research should have a clearly stated and enforced policy addressing the security of records, how identifiers will be handled, and the eventual disposition of records.**

This policy should reflect the law in the jurisdiction and the institution's or agency's own standards. It should be widely distributed and explained to all staff members. Even when guardians of records and identifiers are conscientious and well-intentioned, precautions must be taken against the possibilities of inadvertent or malicious misuse of this information.

Recommendation 10: **Researchers should resist subpoenas that seek the compulsory disclosure of identifiable information.**

While current safeguards are not fully adequate and will require legislative and regulatory change, they do provide researchers with grounds for resisting efforts to force the disclosure of research records with personally identifiable information. Courts are likely to view such resistance more favorably if, from the beginning of the project, the researcher has placed a high value on the confidentiality of the material being collected, has set up stringent safeguards for its protection, and has assured subjects that their data will be kept confidential.

Recommendation 11: **In order to protect fully the confidentiality of research subjects in AIDS studies, administrative and statutory safeguards should be created at federal and state levels to prevent both unjustifiable voluntary and involuntary disclosure of personally identifiable data.**

Such protections ought to be extended to all AIDS research supported by the federal government or to research carried out in institutions receiving federal funds. At the state level, regulatory and statutory protections of the confidentiality of research records ought to be at least as stringent as those adopted by the federal government.

Recommendation 12: **At both federal and state levels the unjustified disclosure of research records by those responsible for their protection and the obtaining of these records under false pretenses or theft should be prohibited by statute and subject to legal sanction.**

At present the protection of research records for AIDS studies depends too heavily upon the professional discretion of those within public agencies or in private research settings. Though the professional integrity of those responsible for the protection of the confidentiality of such records is critical and is supported by codes of professional ethics, it cannot be the sole basis for protecting these records from unwarranted examination. Administrative and statutory safeguards are necessary to provide researchers and administrators with a legal basis for resisting compelled disclosure. Such safeguards are also necessary to protect subjects from unwarranted disclosures by researchers acting without the pressure of compulsion from public or private agencies.

Recommendation 13: **The confidentiality of AIDS research records should not be compromised in the course of program audit and evaluations.**

Because of the special importance of protecting the confidentiality of AIDS research records, it is advisable to strip personal identifiers from all records to be reviewed for audit and evaluation purposes. Though such a requirement may well present difficulties for researchers and some additional burden for auditors and evaluators, we believe that the importance of protecting the privacy of the subjects of AIDS research provides sufficient justification.

Information disclosed for audit purposes should be used only for audit and should not be redisclosed or used against the subject in any other way.

To the extent that it is necessary for auditors to know the identity of individuals to do their job adequately (for example, to verify that subjects in drug trials are not fictitious), decisions about disclosure of such information ought to be made on a case-by-case basis. Strict regulations prohibiting the redisclosure of identifiable information should govern the practice of those conducting audits and evaluations.

Recommendation 14: **Jurisdictions that mandate reporting of AIDS cases should adopt stringent safeguards against subpoena of such records.**

The mandated reporting of AIDS cases places a special responsibility upon public health departments to guarantee the inviolability of the confidential information conveyed by physicians and other health care providers. Without a special statutory provision, like that adopted by the New York City Board of Health, the existence of publicly held records of AIDS cases will pose an undue risk to the privacy rights of persons with AIDS and may subject them to governmental action harmful to their interests.

IX. What Standards Should Institutional Review Boards Follow?

Recommendation 15: **Every AIDS research protocol involving human subjects should receive full review by an Institutional Review Board (IRB), whether or not the research is federally funded.**

Federal regulations governing human subjects research provide the minimum standards for IRB review and encourage institutions to develop more stringent safeguards when appropriate (45 C.F.R. 46.103b). In this spirit, these guidelines are intended to enhance the level of protection.

Federal regulation and institutional practice have developed many ways to reduce the workload of IRBs and to confine their deliberations to protocols that present ethical problems. We believe that, by definition, AIDS research protocols fall into the category that requires review by a full review board.

Research involving survey or interview procedures is exempt from federal regulations, unless *all* of the following conditions exist: "(i) responses are recorded in such a manner that the human subjects can be identified, directly or through identifiers linked to the subjects; (ii) the subject's responses, if they became known outside the research, could reasonably place the subject at risk of criminal or civil liability or be damaging to the subject's financial standing or employability, and (iii) the research deals with sensitive aspects of the subjects own behavior, such as illegal conduct, drug use, sexual behavior, or use of alcohol" (45 CFR section 46.101 (3)). AIDS research using identifiers meets these criteria; therefore, it should not be exempt from review.

Research activities involving no more than minimal risk *and* in which the only involvement of human subjects will be in one or more of a list of categories (such as collection of blood samples by venipuncture, and the study of existing data, documents, records, pathological specimens, or diagnostic specimens) may, under federal regulations, be reviewed through expedited review procedures—that is, review and approval by the IRB chairperson or a subcommittee, without being presented to the full committee—(45 CFR 46.110). However, because of the special problem of confidentiality in AIDS research, all research activities involve more than minimal risk of social harms to the subject and should be given full, not expedited review.

Recommendation 16: **IRBs should consider the concerns about and perceptions of risk held by the subject population.**

The group that considered these guidelines disagreed about whether it is the investigator's responsibility, or the IRB's, to consult with subject populations. Some maintained that IRBs should not consult with subjects themselves but should only encourage investigators in AIDS research to do so. Others felt that, just as IRBs consult outside experts in technical fields, they should be free to—or even required to—consult with members of the subject populations whose interests and welfare they are empowered to protect. They maintained that the IRB need not be reconstituted to allow permanent membership; it can invite subject representatives, either to discuss general issues or a particular protocol.

Only if an IRB has a clear understanding of subjects' interests and concerns can it make a responsible evaluation of risk and benefit in a particular protocol. For the purposes of these guidelines, that understanding can be achieved in different ways; the critical point is that the subjects be involved in considering the ethical aspects of the protocol.

Recommendation 17: **An IRB should make sure that an investigator has considered all aspects of confidentiality; taken all prudent steps to protect privacy, including education of all personnel working on the project; and** communicated in clear, simple, and frank language to the subjects the protections that are in place and the risks, if any, that remain.

In addition to its initial review, an IRB has a responsibility under federal regulations for continuing review at intervals appropriate to the degree of risk, but not less often than once a year. As part of this continuing review, the IRB should evaluate the confidentiality protections to determine their adequacy.

X: When Is Consent Required?

Informed consent, derived from the principle of respect for persons, is a cornerstone of the ethical conduct of research with human subjects. These guidelines reaffirm the importance of obtaining informed consent from prospective research subjects but they also recognize that the practice must be modified for certain situations.

Recommendation 18: **Informed consent should be obtained from the human subjects of any research protocol that involves interviews with patients or family, friends, or sexual contacts; or any collection of data that results in identifiable information.**

The basic elements of informed consent in the Code of Federal Regulations (45 C.F.R. 46.116) are a guide in this respect, although not all elements need be present in all protocols. Particularly important are statements that the study involves research and an explanation of its purposes, procedures, and expected duration; a description of any reasonably foreseeable risks or discomforts; a description of any reasonably foreseeable benefits; a statement about confidentiality; an explanation of whom to contact if the subject has questions; and a statement that participation is voluntary and that refusal to participate or decision to withdraw from the protocol will not result in the loss of benefits to which the subject is otherwise entitled.

Recommendation 19: **If a signed consent form is the only way of linking a particular subject to a research protocol, and the principal risk would be potential harm resulting from a breach of confidentiality, an IRB may waive the signing of the consent form, under the provision of 45 C.F.R. 46.117 [c].**

Informed consent must always be obtained; the consent form, which is only documentation of that process, may sometimes be waived.

IRBs might also consider alternatives or additions to signed consent forms retained by the researcher: one alternative is for the researcher to give the subject a written assurance of the confidentiality provisions of the research project.

Recommendation 20: **An IRB may approve research involving only the use of hospital medical records without requiring that investigators obtain in-**

formed consent from each subject as long as that person was notified that medical records may be used for research purposes.

Much epidemiological research is carried out solely through the use of medical records. The ethical problems of such a practice are not completely resolved. Some believe that patients have the right to refuse to have such records used for research without prior consent. Many researchers believe, however, that such an option would unduly impede research without significantly enhancing subjects' privacy. The issue of honoring refusals for the use of medical records in research ought to be considered by IRBs and the continuing advisory board suggested in Section XII.

If an IRB approves research involving medical records, the patient must be protected from any unjustifiable release of information from the medical record, and no identifiers should be used in any publication from the research. In the case of already existing medical records, living patients should be informed (if they can be located) that these records may be used for research purposes, again with appropriate protections. IRBs should also consider carefully the conditions, if any, under which researchers will be permitted to contact for further information subjects whose records they have reviewed.

Recommendation 21: **Although persons with AIDS do not have the right to consent to surveillance in jurisdictions where AIDS is a legally reportable disease, they should be informed about public health reporting.**

To affirm their dignity as individuals and to give them the opportunity to protect their own interests, persons with AIDS should be told what information about them must be reported and what protections are in place to secure the confidentiality of the data. Of course, they retain the right to consent to research.

XI: The Need For Consistency

Recommendation 22: **Legal protections and policies governing confidentiality of research data should be consistent across various legal jurisdictions, research institutions, and public health bodies.**

The rigorous protection of research data should not depend on vagaries of geography, inclination, or individual consciences. To some extent the protections afforded by the federal regulations governing human subjects research are a helpful step toward consistency. But even these regulations are, for good reasons, worded in a general way and are subject to different interpretations by local IRBs.

To encourage consistency, as well as to improve communication, we urge all relevant policy-making bodies to develop a statement about confidentiality, using these guidelines as well as other relevant documents, and to circulate or publish them so that others will be able to compare their own policies. A model statute governing the confidentiality of research data might be developed by, for example, the Commission on Uniform State Laws, as well as a model policy statement for research institutes, public health departments, and so on.

XII: The Need For A Continuing Advisory Board

Recommendation 23: **A continuing advisory board should be established to assess the adequacy of the guidelines' implementation and to provide a forum for discussing issues not now foreseen or encompassed by these guidelines.**

As AIDS research progresses, and new information is developed, new issues in confidentiality will arise. It is important to have a forum in which all those involved can meet to discuss these issues, to represent the interests of their constituents, and to mediate conflicts. Such a board would be made up of representatives of the subject populations, researchers, public health officials, representatives of private agencies, ethicists, and others.

The existence of this group would not preclude the establishment of special advisory groups within other agencies—the National Institutes of Health, for example—to consider particular protocols. However, the purpose of this board would be to take up policy questions and to discuss broad-based issues that arise as research progresses, not to serve as a "super-IRB" reviewing individual protocols. In a specific instance the board could, if asked, offer an advisory opinion on a protocol.

The composition, funding, authority, and accountability of such a board are beyond the scope of these guidelines. However, one possibility would be for various public and private agencies interested in AIDS research cooperatively to set up a board, provide adequate funding, and name members. In that way the individual members could represent the interests of their sponsoring organizations, report to their organizations about the deliberations and the views of other interested groups, and facilitate communication among them. The board should be an advisory body whose recommendations can carry considerable moral and political weight.

XIII: Communication and Education

Recommendation 24: **All those who do research on AIDS must make a commitment to communicate, as fully and frankly as possible, their policies on confidentiality.**

Those who do research on AIDS should candidly explain why certain kinds of information are needed and what protections exist—and perhaps most difficult, what risks about disclosure of data the subject undertakes in entering the study. These risks should be minimized as much as possible, but where they exist, they should be disclosed.

Educational efforts should be undertaken within subject communities to provide up-to-date and accurate information about confidentiality so that potential subjects are neither needlessly alarmed nor unduly complacent about the risks to confidentiality should they become research subjects. Organizations that represent subject interests should also undertake efforts to inform their constituents about these questions.

If AIDS is to be understood and controlled, trust between researcher and subject is essential. We hope that these guidelines will serve to reinforce that trust where it already exists and to create it where it has not existed before.

PART IV
Legal Problems of AIDS Patients and Health Care Providers

Legal Implications of the AIDS Epidemic

Leonard Glantz, J.D.
Associate Director, Boston University School of Public Health
Professor of Health Law, Boston University School
of Public Health and Medicine

It is important to keep in mind the differences between what makes AIDS special and what makes AIDS similar to other conditions and other problems that we have confronted. First, there have been, historically, and will continue to be, perhaps now even more than ever, a conflict between civil liberties and public health legislation. As you know, people who have opposed fluoridation of water continue to oppose fluoridation of water; people who do not want to wear motorcycle helmets or seat belts bring lawsuits to invalidate laws that require them to do so; and police stop cars randomly on the highways to see whether people are drunk while they are driving. These examples reflect the presence of a past and present conflict between civil liberties, personal liberties, and important, mandatory public health measures. What we have always been confronted with is weighing these conflicts to determine whether the personal liberties of individuals outweigh the states' needs or desires to protect the public health.

Second, the state and federal governments have traditionally had great difficulty in regulating areas of uncertainty. There is so much that we do not know about AIDS that it makes it difficult to promulgate useful regulation. Oftentimes, the fact that uncertainty exists makes it desirable for us to have regulations and laws that make people feel more comfortable.

Third, when we use words such as "rights" or "obligation," we need to consider seriously what these words mean. For example, I have heard discussions about the "right" to be a blood donor. It is not clear to me where that right comes from or how one would construe this to be a right. Perhaps it is a privilege of some sort. When we discuss more difficult issues such as discrimination, we must be quite specific about the legal concepts at issue.

Finally, I want to point out that in the absence of a law prohibiting discrimination, discrimination is lawful in the United States. Whether you agree with this as a moral proposition is not the issue. Even with respect to those laws that do prohibit discrimination, there were (and are) many exceptions, especially where a factual basis exists for discriminating against those individuals. For example, in employment discrimination law, the issue of whether the complained of discrimination is lawful has always been whether there is a bona fide occupational requirement that justifies the discrimination. If it is, then an employer can discriminate. The Supreme Court, for example, has held that schools of nursing can reject applicants who are deaf, because being able to hear is considered to be a bona fide occupational requirement for being a nurse.[1]

I would like you to keep all those things, if possible, in your mind as we begin to consider the legal implications of this epidemic.

The Rights of Patients Hospitalized with AIDS

George J. Annas, J.D., M.P.H.
Edward Utley Professor of Health Law
Chief, Health Law Section, Boston University Schools of
Public Health and Medicine

A number of well-respected legal and health care professionals believe that with respect to AIDS, we need to start over again with different rules. Other people would have us adhere to well-defined principles of health and hospital law. I believe we should look at the laws as they currently exist, examine the known facts about AIDS, and apply existing legal tenets to the facts. In most cases, the laws as they relate to patients' rights are quite adequate to protect the AIDS patient, with the possible exception of the area of confidentiality of patient information. In some cases, we are going to experience the tension between the rights of individual patients and the rights of a community confronted with a deadly, contagious disease. Some rights that we take for granted for most patients will not be so easily won or taken for granted in AIDS patients. I use the term "rights" to mean those privileges, privacies, and protections that are easily recognizable and protected by statutes, regulations, and case law.

The concept of patients' rights is of relatively recent origin, still more often seen as an ethical obligation of physicians rather than a legal obligation. It is perhaps still honored more often in discussion than in reality. As an example to remind people that the history of patients' rights is very recent in the history of law, the first important document about patients' rights was prepared after the French Revolution. One of the first public health proclamations made was to limit the number of patients in a hospital bed (two-to-a-bed) in France. Some people have argued that we have not come very far since then. In 1973, the American Hospital Association issued the Patient's Bill of Rights, which is still the model in this country for patients' rights relating to health care providers.[2] In 1975, when I wrote about the rights of hospital patients, I had some very unkind things to say about that Bill of Rights because of its vagueness, lack of specificity, and lack of enforcement mechanisms.[3] It is symbolic that at least the American Hospital Association recognized that patients have rights—that was a step in the right direction. In 1985, the Ethics Committee of the American Hospital Association, which has met regularly for the last two years, had occasion to review all of the policies of the American Hospital Association. They made various recommendations about ethics but also looked at the Patient's Bill of Rights. They thought it was a fine document that did not need to be changed in any way.

In dealing with patients' rights, it is easy to take an otherworldly position and say, "Yes, patients have all these rights; we don't have to worry about it." Patients do not have all these rights. A prime example is confidentiality of medical records. "Confidentiality" in the hospital means that everybody in the hospital except the patient gets to see his medical record. Unfortunately, that is often very true. When we talk about patients' rights, we are talking about a setting where they often do not have them.

First, informed consent is, by far, the most important, well-established patient "right." Before anyone treats you, you have the right to know what he is going to do to you, the right to be informed about the risks (the risks of death or serious bodily disability), information about alternative treatments, and what the major problems of recuperation are likely to be. When an AIDS patient is treated, he should be treated like any other patient in terms of the information that is given to him or her and in terms of what is going to be done. This is an absolute right, supported thoroughly by case law.

Under what circumstances can a patient refuse treatment? For example, if an individual has been diagnosed as having AIDS and has been admitted to the hospital for treatment of pneumonia that he has acquired as a result of his AIDS, does he have the right to refuse treatment for his pneumonia? The patient's pneumonia is said to be treatable. The physicians believe that there is a 50% chance or better that they can treat his pneumonia and that he can go on to live for another year or two until he ultimately succumbs to his disease. The individual in this case said, "I do not want to be treated for the pneumonia." What he was saying specifically was, "If I have AIDS, let me die now; I do not want to go through treatment or living like this for the next year or two." Does the fact that he has AIDS make him somehow different than any other individual? The commentaries about this case in a recent *Hastings Center Report* share three widely differing views.[4] All of the commentators are absolutely convinced that they know the answer; all of the approaches are different. The legal solution to the dilemma is that you cannot be treated without your informed consent. The right to an informed consent is meaningless unless you have the corollary right to act on or refuse to act on the information given to you.

All of us have a problem with people who refuse treatment that could keep them living for a longer period of time. Nevertheless, competent adults have the right to refuse lifesaving or even life-sustaining treatment. The case of William Bartling in California involved a 70-year-old gentleman on a ventilator.[5] He had a number of underlying diseases and asked that the ventilator be disconnected; the hospital refused. It publicly pronounced that it was on the side of life, not of death, and that it was the hospital's obligation to do everything to keep him alive. Unfortunately, it took a California appeals court to say that it is the patient's right to decide whether or not to be treated, not the hospital's right to decide whether or not to treat a patient. Hospitals and doctors have no independent right to treat patients against their will.

The New Jersey Supreme Court in *In the Matter of Conroy* recently opined that the right to refuse treatment even applies to nutrition; competent adults have the right to refuse to be artificially fed.[6] Surely, the right to refuse treatment applies to an AIDS patient, as long as the patient is competent. By competent, we do not mean that a patient agrees with you, that they are not depressed, or that they have the same lifestyle as you. Competence means that a patient understands the nature and consequences of his decision. The patient understands he is sick, the treatment you have proposed, the alternatives, and what may happen if he chooses to receive or not to receive a given course of treatment.[7] Unless you are going to treat AIDS patients differently from every other critically ill person, there is no reason to deny them their right to control their treatment. An AIDS patient has the right to an informed decision, to consent to treatment, and a right to refuse treatment. I think a patient dying from AIDS should have 24-hour-a-day visiting rights, for example, and that they should have all the things you would give to any other patient who is terminally ill. It may be important as well to have patient advocates. For example, the Veterans Administration allows veterans' groups to develop advocacy systems so that veterans can help other veterans in a hospital. The gay and other at-risk communities should continue to develop the AIDS Action Committees to advise and offer counsel to these victims both in and outside of the hospital. The hospitals should not only allow these advocates in the hospital, but actually encourage their participation.[3]

With respect to human experimentation, these patients should be treated as any other patient; that is, you respect their right to fully informed consent, you respect their welfare, their right not to participate, to be free from coercion, their rights of privacy and confidentiality. One can understand why research on an AIDS ward has all the notions of isolation, specialness, and negative stigma, but research has to be done in a way that protects and promotes patients' rights. These issues have to be confronted on an individual and institutional basis.[8]

Finally, I would like to briefly discuss one aspect of the confidentiality issue. In *Tarasoff v. Regents of the University of California*, a psychiatrist was found to have a duty to warn a potential victim that his patient threatened the victim's life in a psychotherapy session.[9] The Supreme Court of California stated that the legal test of liability was whether the psychiatrist knew *or should have known* that his patient would cause harm to a certain person, and indeed did cause harm. I would argue, at present, given the current state of medical knowledge, there is no duty to warn other people (other than a spouse) that a person has a positive test for the HTLV-III antibody. However, if medical data demonstrate that a person is infected with HTLV-III virus and this infectivity is able to be spread to another person who contracts the disease, there may indeed be a burden on the health care practitioner to notify people who are *at risk* of contracting a lethal disease from the infected patient.

In conclusion, the patients' rights issues for AIDS victims are the same as for anyone else. They are entitled to the same rights to informed consent to refuse treatment, to respect for their person, and to the primary rights regarding informed consent and confidentiality.

Quarantine and AIDS

Alvin Novick, M.D.
Professor of Biology, Yale University
President-Elect, American Association of
Physicians for Human Rights

When I chose to focus on the issue of quarantine and the AIDS victim, I believe that I placed my head squarely in the lion's mouth. The topic is outrageously frightening. Soon, it may be both absolutely appropriate and legitimately in the public health interest, at least in some cases, to isolate or restrict the freedom of certain individuals. At the same time, we will face the horrendous reality that by protecting society from these individuals, we may be taking away rights or freedoms from all of us. In the Declaration of Independence, we were endowed with the right of life, liberty, and the pursuit of happiness. I do not yet believe that any other body of law adopted thereafter takes away from us these natural rights.

In June, 1984, legislation was enacted in Connecticut permitting the quarantine of persons with communicable diseases who are judged to be a threat to public health.[10] This legislation was apparently in response to a series of media events which concerned an unfortunate woman in Connecticut who had many vulnerabilities. She was a black woman, allegedly an IV drug user, and a prostitute. In addition, she was ill. After women, IV drug users, prostitutes, and blacks, I believe that patients are among the most vulnerable people in our society. Also among the list of vulnerable people in our community are human research subjects. Medical scientists (that includes me) are perhaps paternalistic by virtue of our training; as such, through education, intellect, stature, and demeanor, we take away from our patients and our research subjects their autonomy. I believe that the Connecticut legislation was enacted in good faith. The statute reads as follows:

> Any town, city or borough director of health may order any person into confinement whom he has reasonable grounds to believe to be infected with any communicable disease . . . and who is unable or unwilling to conduct himself in such manner as to not expose other persons to danger of

infection . . . whenever such action is necessary to protect and preserve the public health.[10]

The extent to which this legislation is currently, or may come to be, applicable to persons with AIDS or related illnesses, or those judged to be carrying or able to transmit the AIDS agent, has not been established. If it is to be applied, procedures must be established that are so sensitive and rational that they can be understood by reasonable people to be necessary, appropriate, respectful, beneficial to persons and to society and fair.

In the not too distant future, we will recognize situations in which there is a legitimate public health interest in controlling infection. We must begin to consider those public interests that on balance will justify restrictions on individual rights. It is well-established in American law and custom that society can restrict the rights of individuals who are demonstrably infectious. A contemporary analysis would also require that no constraints be applied unless they are demonstrably necessary, promise to be effective in protecting society, and are minimally invasive. In terms of AIDS, who may be said to have a communicable disease? Whatever our uncertainties today, and there are many, we may reasonably conjecture that we will have an accurate picture of the course of infection and infectiousness in the next year or two, and that we are likely to have practical access to tests for infectiousness in the future.

I believe that at that point, a realistic assessment of infectiousness will be possible. On the other hand, it will allow people to behave responsibly. If pure, definite evidence of infectiousness is possible, then education is possible. It will also make people legally vulnerable to constraint. We need to know, as researchers and in the manner of basic information, what sexual practices or drug-related practices relate to viral and/or disease transmission. It is not very helpful in this context to know that intimate sexual contact is associated with transmission. We really have to know some details. Those details are embarrassing to our conservative federal government and to investigators. Such survey studies are difficult to perform and the details are not easy to pursue. They are not easy to pursue because no one chooses to fund them and because many are afraid to engage in such research lest it adversely affect a career. There are perhaps many other reasons why that information is not pursued but, lacking that information, we will be severely restricted in designing appropriate constraints.

Not every informed and compassionate physician, patient advocate, scientist or counselor would necessarily agree, on the basis of current data or future data, on the direction that public policy should take. We are experienced enough to know that current data and uncertain future data will be interpreted differently by different interest groups. Even so, we require and will continue to require massive and diverse educational programs nationwide, directed towards the general public, the members of at-risk groups, and at the broad range of health professionals. Such programs must be mounted in each substantial community to ensure knowledgeability that will enable persons to protect themselves and will allow health professionals to provide optimal care and wise advice. Such programs have begun in many communities; in general, however, they are insufficient to meet community needs. Massive professional commitment, publicity, organization, and funding are necessary if the job is to be effective.

If persons with AIDS, AIDS-related illnesses, persons who are antibody positive to HTLV-III, or in the future, all persons who are shown to be infectious by whatever tests we have, if they are to be isolated or quarantined, I maintain that society will be irreparably and permanently damaged. There is historical precedent for isolating certain groups based on danger to society. The internment of the Japanese during World War II was one such example. The *least* invasive method of determining infectivity could be by testing. More invasive methods are rumor, surveillance, and monitoring, invasions of privacy similar to what the Nazis did through the Gestapo. It is not unthinkable. There are certainly communities in our country who would welcome reports of people who are believed to be infectious.

There are even worse scenarios than that. Since it might be difficult to survey the entire American population for antibody positivity, an easy path might be taken to identify people by their social risk group: to identify gay men, IV drug users, hemophiliacs, female sex partners of at-risk men, female sex partners of blood transfusion recipients or of hemophiliacs. No one would seek them out in the upper middle class residential communities of America; they would be sought out in those populations that are more vulnerable than others.

In Texas, an attempt was made to recriminalize homosexual activity such that anyone committing sodomy would be convicted and sent to jail. How often is sodomy witnessed that you were not a partner of unless you participate in group sex? I expect that few occurrences of sodomy, outside of rape, are reported. The thought that it can be controlled through legislation is naive, evil, and most importantly, ineffective.

The most obvious approach that at least offers a possibility of success are rational educational programs directed to those people in the at-risk groups and to any person who appears to be a threat to the community. In those specific cases where a threat is a real one, further sensitive and appropriate counseling should be undertaken until a rational solution is achieved. The cost of counseling to the few who refuse to cooperate with appropriate public health advice would be much less than the quarantine scenarios. Further, the real solution is to decrease the vulnerability of the persons in the AIDS at-risk groups by raising their self-image and society's image of them. We should stop our political, social, and religious leaders from making outrageously unacceptable, bigoted remarks about fine American men and women. We should try to be more effective in reducing these vulnerabilities, and eliminating many of the behaviors that we are concerned about, before we risk the basic political and personal freedoms we enjoy in America.

Comment

(Leonard Glantz): There are quarantine laws in every state in the United States that deal not only with AIDS but with all varieties of infectious diseases. People with tuberculosis or leprosy used to be treated by quarantine. Mental patients are regularly quarantined. People who are dangerous because of their medical condition, or mental condition, are put in locked wards and locked hospitals to protect society. As unhappy a possibility as it is, there is significant precedent for using quarantine in cases of great fear and in cases of infectious diseases.

Disability and Estate Planning Considerations

Steven Ansolabehere, J.D.
Director, AIDS Law Project
Gay and Lesbian Advocates and Defenders
Member, Mayor's Committee on AIDS

I have been engaged in the private practice of law for five years and am Director of the AIDS Law Project. I am gay; my clientele is primarily gay. The lay and professional legal press viewed the AIDS problem as involving young men who die young as single individuals. What does this mean to those people? Thirty-year-old men—at least several new clients each week—were requesting me to prepare their wills. It was an extraordinary thing that I had never seen happen before. Their concerns soon turned not only to wills, but to their legal status in terms of a personal relationship between gay individuals. I was suddenly confronted with gay couples who were concerned about their status as couples, and how to make that status as couples legally enforceable. I think this facet of the problem is an important one for all medical providers. First, gay couples are not a legally recognized entity. Because they are not a legally recognized entity, they cannot inherit from each other; they have no right to each other's Social Security benefits if a partner is disabled; they have no rights of general inheritance; and, they do not have the favorable presumption under the law to be appointed a conservator or guardian, as a married person would, in the event of such disability. There are ways in which those contingencies, through wills and powers of attorney, may be provided for. These are some of the legal services that a gay legal practitioner provides to his other gay clients. If you are a medical practitioner and have an AIDS patient who has a lover, then you should be sensitive to some important legal issues that relate to your patient. The patient's lover can be named legally as the person to whom all questions regarding treatment should be referred. Ordinarily, issues of medical treatment are left to the patient and his or her next of kin. It is now possible for such patients to legally have their lovers named as next of kin, for all intents and purposes, if they are aware of this possible approach.

Approximately two years ago, I volunteered to work for Gay and Lesbian Advocates and Defenders (GLAD) in a role dealing with AIDS discrimination. The first case that came to my attention, and to GLAD's attention, was a Boston-area hospital that was admitting patients in high risk groups and placing them on blood or hepatitis precautions. The implications of this decision to gay men who were being admitted (openly gay men, in any case) was that if they were admitted, for example, with a broken leg to this hospital, the nurses, physicians, and staff would approach him with masks, gloves, gowns, and other paraphernalia, even though they had no symptoms of AIDS and were completely asymptomatic. We do not know how long or how actively this policy was pursued. Obviously, it is very difficult to know who is gay and who is not gay. The policy did not make any sense; the hospital administration quickly reversed its policy and adjusted its activities accordingly.

Later, we experienced a lull in legal issues brought to GLAD's attention. We were expecting an explosion of discrimination cases based on media reports and the high anxiety levels that seemed to be prevailing throughout the gay and straight community. This "explosion" was not seen at that time.

The concerns that were brought to us were by gay men who were seeing their physicians about what the patient thought were symptoms of AIDS. Ironically, their concerns were not whether they would be identified as having AIDS. Their concerns related to the confidentiality of their medical records. They did not want their records to fall into the wrong hands, revealing that they were gay. One example involved an employee who worked for an insurance company. Because he worked for a health insurance company, his insurance was through that same company. He was worried about seeing his physician. If he admitted that he was gay and had serious concerns about having AIDS, he thought that any information transmitted to his physician would reach his employer, as his employer was the insurer. There is simply no way to safeguard this type of medical record. The only way I know of is to be treated by a physician you know well who will take efforts to safeguard your confidentiality. As I think all health care providers will admit, medical records are anything but confidential. Within any given facility, those records are available to any person so requesting the records.

On a national basis, there is no uniform law which prohibits discrimination. On a state by state basis, however, many legislatures have passed laws that ban discrimination based upon race, sex, national origin, or creed. Recently, almost all of the state legislatures have adopted prohibitions against discrimination based upon disability. These prohibitions against discrimination of the disabled are the primary tools that AIDS rights attorneys or civil rights attorneys are using to protect their clients against discrimination.

One discrimination case involved a physician seeing patients with AIDS in a co-op housing unit in New York.[11] The co-op attempted to evict the physician. He sought judicial relief and was defended not only by the Lambda Legal Defense Fund but also by the State Attorney General. To my knowledge, this is the first time that a State Attorney General has found it necessary to join a suit on the side of the discriminated-against, disabled party. The basis of that suit was a state law forbidding discrimination based upon disability. As you know, discrimination, in general, is not forbidden in the United States. You may discriminate against me, for example, because I am gay, because I have green eyes, or I am balding, or any number of other reasons that may seem irrational or baseless, but you have the right to do so. You do not have the right to discriminate against me when there is a specific statutory provision prohibiting you from doing so.

I would also like to point out several of the cases that have arisen under these disability statutes. One of these cases involved two flight attendants employed by United Airlines who operated out of Chicago. Both of them had enlarged lymph nodes and were known to be gay by their co-employees; therefore, they were suspected of having AIDS. Fellow employees objected to their continuing to work flights, and, specifically, objected to their handling food for the flying customer. United Airlines dismissed them. The case went to arbitration; the arbitrator awarded the flight attendants back pay and ordered United to reinstate them. The arbitrator decided that United had failed to prove that it was medically impermissible for these people to fulfill their jobs; that is, to prove that at least one of the attendants had AIDS. The question presented did not involve whether a person with AIDS can be fired, but rather what medical proof exists that shows his condition causes dangers either to himself or to others (persons to whom he is serving food, for example) and prevents him from performing his tasks. Is he a danger to others? The burden of proof was placed on United to show that he was a danger to the flying passengers, to the other members of the crew, or to himself. The arbitrator found they had failed on all counts.

Similar litigation is going on now in Florida. Two county employees had been fired because they have been diagnosed as having AIDS.[12] The county in question had passed legislation forbidding the employment of any person who has AIDS. That case is still being litigated.

Another case, *Doe v. Charlotte Memorial Hospital*, involves a nurse in North Carolina who has been diagnosed as having AIDS. He was first assigned to a nonpatient contact position, with his permission and acquiescence. Later, he was fired altogether, primarily because he has AIDS. This matter is also still in litigation.

Locally, we have a number of problems and issues that we have dealt with in a similar vein. The AIDS Action Committee has only one lawsuit outstanding.

Until recently, most employers have chosen not to discriminate. At present, however, the level of discrimination is growing enormously.

What we are beginning to see is people who do not care to consider relevant facts about the disease. They refuse to discuss the issues with the AIDS Action Committee or with anyone else. They seem to consider the data about relative risks to themselves or to others coming in contact with employees, patients or tenants with AIDS to be irrelevant. In Boston, we have one suit against a local dentist who has flatly refused to treat any AIDS patients regardless of whether they have any other contagious disabilities. It was enough for that dentist to discover that the patient had AIDS in order to decide that he would not treat such persons.

In contrast, we have a local alcohol rehabilitation hospital that had adopted a policy that no AIDS patients would be allowed in the hospital. Their argument was that they lacked the proper facilities to treat an AIDS patient. They were not willing to inquire into whether, in fact, an AIDS patient required special facilities. When we contacted their general counsel, an agreement was worked out between my organization and that hospital. They agreed to examine each individual AIDS patient as he applied for admission to determine whether he was, in fact, someone who should not be there on the basis of his disability, whether he posed a risk to others, or whether the hospital setting posed a risk to the patient due to inadequate facilities.

In the AIDS discrimination area, we want a policy forbidding blanket discrimination. What we insist on is that each case be considered individually. Every AIDS patient does not need to be isolated. Every AIDS patient is not contagious. In general, litigation is a poor tool; however, I think it is the only one we have left.

In general, health care providers in Boston have been superb in their efforts to be concerned about the civil rights and liberties of their patients. In fact, they have far exceeded any expectations I could have had. At the same time, we are beginning to see a willingness of people to believe that they have an absolute right, a moral right, to protect themselves from this contagion—not only to protect themselves from the contagion but to remain ignorant as to what their risk is. People seem determined that they have the right to say, "I will not look at this person, I won't deal with him." This perspective is very difficult to confront and it is one we are trying to prevent.

The Right to Receive Health Care

Michael Callen
Co-Founder, Gay Men with AIDS
Founding Member, People With AIDS
Member, New York State AIDS Advisory Council

As public health, public safety, and other health professionals become more exposed to patients with AIDS, the manner in which they fulfill their professional obligations vary, depending on their own sense of professionalism and duty. As an example, I was called recently by the New York City Commission on Human Rights. The Commission had received a number of complaints from social workers who said that they were not able to arrange for ambulances to transport people with AIDS either to or from the hospital. The Commission asked our organization, Gay Men with AIDS, if we would call the ambulance companies and request an appointment for an ambulance or ambulettes. The excuse we used was that on a given date, we needed to be driven to the hospital for chemotherapy. In all instances, we were given an appointment. Only after we had a confirmed appointment did we mention casually that we had AIDS. In several instances, our appointments were cancelled on the spot and we were told "We don't take people with AIDS. We don't transport them." These comments raised some very interesting legal issues. Some of these companies were sued; others settled quickly before their cases proceeded to litigation. In one case that has not settled, the issues concern whether there is a difference between ambulances and ambulettes. A company that provides ambulance services is required to take emergency patients whenever they are called. People who have received chemotherapy, as is the case with many people who have AIDS, do not need the more elaborate (and more expensive) services of an ambulance. They need an ambulette, which is a van that can pick up more than one person, with some medical services available. It is less expensive. The ambulette company argued that they will not carry people with AIDS because other patients in the ambulette would not ride with people who have AIDS. What would happen, they asked, if, after chemotherapy, a person with AIDS vomits and someone gets AIDS from their vomitus? Or if they bleed in the ambulette? Would the ambulance company be liable? Because the law is not clear, and because of paranoia, some people with AIDS receiving treatment with chemotherapy get to the hospital by the more expensive means, an ambulance. Of course, most people ignore their severe discomfort and take the subway or taxicabs.

Health insurance is another serious issue. Soon, gay men may be an uninsurable class. Insurance companies that have access to our medical records can identify trends by the treatments administered. Gay men are beginning to become very nervous if they have a history of treatment for sexually transmitted diseases, amoebic diseases, or T-cell abnormalities. Will these data be used as presumptive evidence of membership in a high risk group? Are the data going to be used to cancel policies?

Several dentists refused to see me after my diagnosis of AIDS. I believe that there are many health care professionals who do not want to treat or examine patients with AIDS. When I spoke with a spokesperson for the American Medical Association, I was told that while individual hospitals may bring disciplinary actions against their employees and physicians, hospitals are allowed, in general, to police themselves. Thus, a physician or a nurse can refuse to offer non-emergency treatment to hospitalized or other patients unless hospital policy expressly forbids such discrimination.

Another area of serious concern relates to the use of a quarantine to address the public health risks of AIDS. I do not actually believe that quarantine is likely to happen soon—we know, however, that the issue has been discussed at high levels in government. In Connecticut, for example, we attempted to address the question of quarantine before the Connecticut legislation. We were not prepared to say that quarantine is never effective. We were not prepared to challenge the concept that states have the right, in certain instances, to quarantine people. Almost every state has quarantine legislation. What was unusual about the situation in Connecticut is that the legislature was actually adding a 72-hour review process in an attempt to provide a right of appeal for the infected person. Three independent professionals must recommend quarantine before such an order may be issued.

I am aware of some people with AIDS who continue to have sex. Most, of course, vigorously practice safer sex—to protect themselves and their partners; a minority, however, practice unsafe sex. A number of researchers are very concerned because they ask their research subjects questions about sexual activities. Occasionally, some people with AIDS admit that they are continuing to have sex with people who are unaware of the fact that the person with AIDS is ill. A number of the researchers feel very troubled about whether they should disclose these facts to the local health departments or to take other action on an individual basis. It is here that tension is the greatest. It must be quite frustrating to reconcile that a patient has AIDS and may be exposing his sexual partners to AIDS and other sexually transmitted diseases. We cannot address this issue yet, because of the state of the scientific art. It is appropriate, however, to continue to address and reason through these very complicated and painful issues, because sooner, rather than later, they will be upon us.

Question

It is my understanding of the epidemiology of this disease that an individual who has AIDS and still engages in unsafe sexual activities may be potentially less infectious than a person without symptoms but HTLV-III positive. There are data that suggest it was harder to retrieve the live virus from the saliva of individuals with AIDS than patients with infection but without active disease. The scientific construct would be that people with AIDS might have fewer target cells left by the time they develop symptoms. If this is taken as a premise, then the problem becomes a more generalized one. In terms of the provider–patient relationship, people who are at risk should be told that behavior modification has great significance for the individual to avoid exposing themselves to the virus that might be deleterious both to themselves and to the general community. I think we should not want to further victimize individuals, further adding to the stigma. The public is relying on us to be honest—we do not know who is infectious, given the technologies available to us at present. We believe that individuals with AIDS are clearly in a high risk group; however, are they more at risk for spreading contagion than many other gay people who do not have clinical symptoms? We do not know the answer at this time.

Answer

This is an often quoted perspective that people with AIDS like to discuss. For a while, physicians were beginning to suggest that we may be the safest people to have sex with and that it is actually the asymptomatic clone who may be carrying the putative causative agent. Irrespective of the realities of the science, people tend to agree that everyone, especially those people with AIDS, have an ethical obligation to apprise potential sex partners of their health status. Researchers do not quite know what to say about sexual contacts with a person with AIDS. How should he be sexually active? Where do you draw the line, legally and ethically, in the absence of being able to establish who is contagious, and when and how a person should abstain?

Question

(Leo Murphy, New England Hemophilia Association): The hemophiliac's problems with AIDS are characterized by an apparently complete lack of confidentiality. Every place of employment knows who their hemophiliac is. Because of this, no hemophiliac can get health "insurance," as it is traditionally structured. I am a freelance contractor. Because people know that I have hemophilia they won't hire me, primarily because virtually 100% of all hemophiliacs test positive for the HTLV-III virus. This presents a very difficult situation.

Answer

We do tend to be risk group chauvinists. While the issues in the gay population may be more vocally framed, they are no more important than the issues for other at-risk groups.

Question

(Harvey Barton, M.D.): I have a question regarding legal aspects of reporting HTLV-III antibody positivity. If an insurance company or legal entity submits a subpoena to a researcher (M.D. or Ph.D), does he or she have to report the results of laboratory data, physical exam, or medical history information that would place someone in an at-risk group—especially if they are HTLV-III antibody positive, or if they have altered T-cell lymphocyte helper–suppressor ratios? Is that individual required to report those results to insurance companies, or to the courts if the medical records are subpoenaed?

Answer

In general, when a person applies for insurance, he signs a waiver with the insurance carrier that permits the carrier complete access to his medical records. If in fact the patient signed the waiver, and the insurance company presents it to you, I think you have the same responsibility to deliver the records as you would if the patient himself said, "I want to see my records." The patient could rescind the consent to release of the records. However, if he did so, he most probably would enable the company to escape payment for his medical bill. There are a number of groups that have argued that the preprinted release forms are not really informed consent because people do not have a choice in deciding whether to release the records—if they want insurance, they sign the form.

I tend to deal with insurance company questions in the same manner as someone deals with interrogatories; that is, try not to answer them. If the insurance question is whether someone suffers from a disease, does the HTLV-III antibody positively constitute a disease? You are the physician—exercise your judgment as to whether it does. If the insurance company asks specific questions, the questions have to be answered truthfully and thoughtfully.

Question

(Cathy Kogger, Mount Sinai Hospital, New York): Please specify what "quarantine" involves. If an AIDS patient is quarantined, would it be for the rest of his life?

Answer

If the Connecticut quarantine legislation were to be applied today, I cannot comprehend a rationale to justify the later release of a quarantined person. Currently, we have no way of proving that a person is not carrying and thus is not able to transmit the HTLV-III virus and the infection. In my opinion, once a person suspected of having or diagnosed as having AIDS is quarantined, the only release from quarantine would be death. When patients with typhoid were placed in quarantine, those people remained in quarantine until there were no more bacilli in their stool samples. If they became noninfectious, they were released. If they remained infectious, they stayed in quarantine.

Question

(Sheldon Landesman, M.D.): With respect to the confidentiality of medical records, at Downstate Medical Center we have attempted to be very careful to separate the medical records of patients from the research data collected on these patients. Sometimes, the legal protections afforded to our research participants are greater than the protections for patients. We try to keep all of our sensitive information out of the medical records. Am I correct in assuming that, in fact, with our Assurance of Confidentiality from the federal government, those research records are more difficult to successfully get at than routine medical records?

Answer

My understanding is that the Assurance of Confidentiality has its legal origin at the National Institute of Alcoholism and Drug Abuse. That institute is interested in collecting information on activities that are illegal. In order to encourage participants to admit to this information, the participants are assured that the information secured by and collated by the researchers cannot be subpoenaed or possessed by other agencies. Similar assurances in the AIDS research area have been granted. In the area of child abuse, for example, if parents who are alcoholics and child abusers who are in research studies involving detoxification and counseling mention in treatment that "I just beat my kid," how does one deal with the state statute that requires the physician to report child abuse? I think that the federal government's position is that one can disclose the incident of child abuse without disclosing any information about the data collated for the study, which is not required to be produced in response to a subpoena.

Question

We will be screening very large populations of blood donors with the ELISA test. Presumably, 0.3% of these donors will be HTLV-III antibody positive. In addition, a data bank of donors who donated to a particular blood donation center will be available in the blood bank's records. What are the current rights of the recipients of such blood donations from people who are identified as HTLV-III positive? Are they to be informed? What are the obligations of the blood centers to those people?

Answer

(Johanna Pindyck, M.D.): Projects are underway to notify patients who have received blood that was potentially contaminated. It is policy evolving toward a recognition that people who have been the recipients of blood from donors who were positive for anti-HTLV-III antibody will probably be told. In addition, there is a National Transfusion Safety Study ongoing, sponsored by the National Heart, Lung, and Blood Institute, the New York Blood Center, and blood centers in Miami, San Francisco, and Los Angeles. We will be testing blood from consenting donors that has been stored prior to the availability of testing and doing prospective follow-ups on recipients in order to define the health implications of contaminated blood.

References

1. *Southeastern Community College v. Davis*, 442 U.S. 397 (1979).
2. American Hospital Association. 1973. A patient's bill of rights. Publication no. 2415.
3. Annas, G.J. 1975. *The rights of hospital patients.* New York: Avon Books.
4. If I have AIDS, then let me die now. 1984. *Hastings Center Report* 14(1): 23–26.
5. *Bartling v. Superior Ct.*, 163 App. 3d 186, 202 Cal. Rptr. 220 (1984).
6. *In the Matter of Conroy*, 98 N.J. 321, 486 A.2d 1209 (1985).
7. Annas, G.J., and J.E. Densberger. 1984. Competence to refuse medical treatment: autonomy vs. paternalism. *Toledo Law Review* 15:561.
8. Annas, G.J., L.H. Glantz, and B.F. Katz. 1977. *Informed consent to human experimentation: the sub-*
   ject's dilemma. Cambridge, MA: Ballinger.
9. *Tarasoff v. Regents of the University of California*, 131 Cal. Rptr. 14, P.2d 334 (1976).
10. Connecticut General Assembly. 1984 Connecticut Acts 84-336. Amending section 19a-2212; an act concerning quarantine measures.
11. *People of the State of New York v. 49 W. 12th St. Tenants Corp.*, No., 43604/83, New York Supreme Court, 1983 (Gammerman); *New York Law Journal* (October 17, 1983):1.
12. *Shuttleworth v. Broward County Office of Budget and Management Policy*, No. 85-0624 (December 11, 1985); *BNA Daily Labor Report* No. 242:E1–E6 (December 17, 1985).

Appendix
Connecticut Quarantine Statute
CONFINEMENT OF PERSONS WITH COMMUNICABLE DISEASE OR HARBORING RADIOACTIVE MATERIAL—HEARINGS
Substitute House Bill No. 5906
Public Act No. 84-336

An act concerning quarantine measures and the reporting of accidental poisonings to the University of Connecticut Health Center.

Be it enacted by the Senate and House of Representatives in General Assembly convened:

Section 1. Section 19a-221 of the general statutes is repealed and the following is substituted in lieu thereof:

(a) For the purposes of this section, (1) "communicable disease" means a disease or condition, the infectious agent of which may pass or be carried, directly or indirectly, from the body of one person or animal to the body of another person or animal; and (2) "respondent" means a person ordered confined under this section.

(b) Any town, city or borough director of health may order any person into confinement whom he has reasonable grounds to believe to be infected with any communicable disease and any person who intentionally or unintentionally harbors in or on the body amounts or radioactive material sufficient to constitute a radiation hazard to others and who is unable or unwilling to conduct himself in such manner as to not expose other persons to danger of infection or irradiation whenever such action is necessary to protect or preserve the public health.

(c) The order by the director shall be in writing setting forth: (1) the name of the person to be confined, (2) the basis for the director's belief that the person has a communicable disease or harbors radioactive material, that the person poses a substantial threat to the public health and that confinement is necessary to protect or preserve the public health, (3) the period of time during which the order shall remain effective, (4) the place of confinement as designated by the director, and (5) such other terms and conditions as may be necessary to protect and preserve the public health. Such order shall also inform the person confined that he has the right to consult an attorney, the right to a hearing under this section, and that if such a hearing is requested, he has the right to be represented by counsel, and that counsel will be provided at the state's expense if he is unable to pay for such counsel. A copy of the order shall be given to such person within twenty-four hours of the issuance of the order, the director of health shall notify the commissioner of health services that such an order has been issued. The order shall be effective for not more than fifteen days, provided further orders of confinement pursuant to this section may be issued as to any respondent for successive periods of not more than fifteen days if issued before the last business day of the preceding period of confinement.

(d) A person ordered confined under this section shall be confined in a place designated by the director of health until such time as such director determines such person no longer poses a substantial threat to the public health or is released by order of a court of competent jurisdiction. Any person who desires treatment by prayer or spiritual means without the use of any drugs or material remedies, but through the use of the principles, tenets or teachings of any church incorporated under chapter 598, may be so treated during his confinement in such place.

(e) A person confined under this section shall have the right to a court hearing and, if such person or his representative requests a hearing in writing, such hearing shall be held within seventy-two hours of receipt of such request, excluding Saturdays, Sundays and legal holidays. A request for a hearing shall not stay the order of confinement issued by the director of health under this section. The hearing shall be held to determine if (1) the person ordered confined is infected with a communicable disease or harbors radioactive material, (2) the person poses a substantial threat to the public health, and (3) confinement of the person is necessary and the least restrictive alternative to protect and preserve the public health. The commissioner of health services shall have the right to be made a party to the proceedings.

(f) Jurisdiction shall be vested in the court of probate for the district in which such person resides or is confined. The probate court administrator shall appoint a three-judge court from among the several judges of probate to conduct the hearing. Such three-judge court shall consist of at least one judge who is an attorney-at-law admitted to practice in this state. The judge of the court of probate having jurisdiction under the provisions of this section shall be a member, provided such judge may disqualify himself in which case all three members of such court shall be appointed by the probate court administrator. Such three-judge court when convened shall be subject to all of the provisions of law as if it were a single-judge court. The involuntary confinement of a person under this section shall not be ordered by the court without the vote of at least two of the three judges convened hereunder. The judges of such court shall designate a chief judge from among their members. All records for any case before the three-judge court shall be maintained in the court of probate having jurisdiction over the matter as if the three-judge court had not been appointed.

(g) Notice of the hearing shall be given the respondent and shall inform him that he or his representative has a right to be present at the hearing; that he has a right to counsel; that he, if indigent or otherwise unable to pay for or obtain counsel, has a right to have counsel appointed to represent him; and that he has a right to cross-examine witnesses testifying at the hearing. If the court finds such respondent is indigent or otherwise unable to pay for or obtain counsel, the court shall appoint counsel for him, unless such respondent refuses counsel and the court finds that the respondent understands the nature of his refusal. The court shall provide such respondent a reasonable opportunity to select his own counsel to be appointed by the court. If the respondent does not select counsel or if counsel selected by the respondent refuses to represent him or is not available for such representation, the court shall appoint counsel for the respondent from a panel of attorneys admitted to practice in this state provided by the probate court administrator in accordance with regulations promulgated by the probate court administrator in accordance with section 45-4d. The reasonable compensation of appointed counsel for a person who is indigent or otherwise unable to pay for counsel shall be established by, and paid from funds appropriated to, the judicial department.

(h) Prior to such hearing, such respondent or his counsel, shall be afforded access to all records including, without limitation, hospital records if such respondent is hospitalized. If such respondent is hospitalized at the time of the hearing, the hospital shall make available at such hearing for use by the patient or his counsel all records in its possession relating to the condition of the respondent. Nothing herein shall prevent timely objection to the admissibility of evidence in accordance with the rules of civil procedure.

(i) At such hearing, the director of health who ordered the confinement of the respondent shall have the burden of showing by clear and convincing evidence that the respondent is infected with a communicable disease or harbors radioactive material and poses a substantial threat to the public health and that confinement of the respondent is necessary and the least restrictive alternative to protect and preserve the public health.

(j) If the court, on such hearing, finds by clear and convincing evidence that the respondent is infected with a communicable disease or harbors radioactive material and poses a substantial threat to the public health and that confinement of the respondent is necessary and the least restrictive alternative to protect and preserve the public health, it shall order (1) the continued confinement of the respondent under such terms and conditions as it deems appropriate until such time as it is determined that his release would not constitute a substantial threat to the public health, or (2) the release of the respondent under such terms and conditions as it deems appropriate to protect the public health.

(k) If the court, on such hearing, fails to find that the conditions required for an order for confinement have been proven, it shall order the immediate release of the respondent.

(l) A respondent may, at any time, move the court to terminate or modify an order made under subsection (1) of this section, in which case a hearing shall be held in accordance with this section. The court shall annually, upon its own motion, hold a hearing to determine if the conditions which required the confinement or restriction of the respondent still exist. If the court, at a hearing held upon motion of the respondent or its own motion, fails to find that the conditions which required confinement or restriction still exist, it shall order the immediate release of the respondent. If the court finds that such conditions still exist but that a different remedy is appropriate under this section, the court shall modify its order accordingly.

(m) Any person aggrieved by an order of the court of probate under this section may appeal to the superior court.

(Section 2 covers procedures for dealing with persons with communicable tuberculosis who leave chronic disease hospitals against medical advice. It has been omitted here.)

Sec. 3. Section 19a-260 of the general statutes is repealed and the following is substituted in lieu thereof:

Any person committed to a chronic disease or isolation hospital under the provisions of section *19a-221,* as amended by Section 1 of this act, who leaves before the termination of the period of commitment may be apprehended by any officer authorized to serve criminal process, and the written request of the superintendent or medical officer of such hospital shall be sufficient warrant for such apprehension.

(Section 4 covers the responsibilities of the University of Connecticut Health Center in reporting accidental poisonings; section 5 repeals certain related sections of the general statutes. These sections have been omitted here.)

Approved June 4, 1984.

Part V
The Impact of AIDS on the Patient, Family, Friends, and Community

Psychiatric Illness in Patients with AIDS

Joseph Barbuto, M.D.
Psychiatrist, New York City
Fellow, Psychiatry Service, Memorial Sloan-
Kettering Cancer Center
Clinical Instructor in Psychiatry,
Cornell University Medical Center

As a practicing psychiatrist in New York City and through my work at the Memorial Sloan-Kettering Medical Center, I have had the opportunity to consult on or have had in treatment approximately 50 patients with AIDS. First, I will attempt to identify what I believe to be the significant social and psychological pressures that a patient with AIDS confronts. Next, I will briefly describe our experience on the psychiatry service at Memorial Hospital with treating AIDS patients, and describe to you some of the psychiatric complications that are apparent.

The AIDS epidemic is having a profound impact on society. It is engendering dramatic social, political, and economic response. The magnitude of this response is largely due to the disastrous medical course and the attendant poor prognosis for the patient. Society has responded to AIDS by creating an atmosphere in which patients find it especially difficult to cope; apparently, AIDS has taken on the aura of a new leprosy in our society. Some of the societal biases against people with other illnesses, such as tuberculosis and cancer, are now inflicted on people with AIDS.

In the political arena, considerable deliberation by government agencies and politicians has been necessary to determine our government's course of action against this epidemic. These delays have been increasingly frustrating for both patients and health caregivers. Economically, the disease has created a new pool of recipients of public assistance because of the extraordinary medical costs and the patient's lack of ability to continue employment as the disease progresses. Finally, AIDS has affected medicine, raising questions for researchers as to the cause of the disease, its mode of transmission, and the development of effective, appropriate treatments. The epidemic has affected medicine further in that it is a serious drain on hospital resources and staff due to the profound severity of the associated illnesses and opportunistic infections. Isolation precautions have been confusing at times for both the medical staff and for patients. Laboratory and intensive or special care resources have been stretched to their physical and economic limits, not to mention the profound toll that working with seriously ill, young, AIDS patients takes on the hospital staff.

As you can imagine, the patient who is diagnosed as having AIDS is subject to significant and complex psychological stresses. Typically, AIDS strikes a young, socially aware, highly intelligent group of people. Our AIDS patients are much more knowledgeable about their illness, new modes of treatment, and prognosis than any other patients facing life-threatening illness. They are aware that carrying this diagnosis represents a serious threat to life. This awareness is made more profound if they know people who have died from AIDS. Patients are constantly vulnerable to infection; they worry about this unique susceptibility constantly. Also, their own self-worth and sense of themselves as carriers of the AIDS virus is always present and pressing.

Isolation, both physical and emotional, is experienced soon after the diagnosis is confirmed. Respiratory and gastrointestinal infections effect a prolonged separation from others. Hospitalized patients are admitted to private rooms with rare visits from family and friends; in some cases, gowns, gloves, and masks are often worn by hospital personnel who care for these patients. Each personal contact is brief. A sense of isolation may also prevail because patients consider themselves to be AIDS carriers and they may even avoid social contacts. In addition, since some have engaged only in anonymous sex, they find themselves alone and bereft of intimate relationships during their illness.

In some cases, the AIDS diagnosis has meant that people who concealed their homosexuality are forced to reveal their lifestyle, notwithstanding their personal preference. Because the illness strikes very specific populations, family members and friends are quickly confronted with the habits and sexual preferences of the patient who may have kept them well-hidden until the onset of the illness. As well, many patients experience the onset of AIDS as a second coming-out; that is, they compare the onset of the illness experientially to the time in their lives when they announced themselves as being gay.

With respect to guilt feelings it is important to remember that, in general, patients with cancer speculate whether they "caused" their illness, perhaps by smoking cigarettes, eating an improper diet, or involvement in certain excesses in lifestyle. AIDS patients similarly experience self-blame over "living life in the fast lane" with multiple, frequent sex partners, illegal drug use, or poor nutritional habits. There are those who have been in long-term monogamous relationships who experience guilt because they believe they incurred the illness by having been unfaithful.

Patients experience a loss of self-esteem in that there is a loss of bodily function, bodily integrity, and appearance. The loss of the ability to sustain a career or to participate in social, sexual, and loving relationships also diminish self-esteem. A dimunition in the available modes of pleasure and gratification heighten that sense of low self-esteem.

Dependence is both real and feared. Imagine a man in his mid–30s who is abruptly converted into a geriatric-like patient with debilitation, medical constriction, and the inability to focus on and perceive activities of daily living without the help of others.

Concerns over appearance are commonplace. The lesions of Kaposi's sarcoma are raised and purple in color and appear anywhere on the body. When they appear on the face, marked distortions in appearance are observed. Herpes lesions and oral candidiasis affect appearance as well. Chemotherapy and radiation therapy for tumors associated with AIDS have their own dramatic effects on appearance.

The financial strain becomes overwhelming for all persons, even wealthy patients, with this illness. As infections occur and recur, medical bills mount. There are recurring hospitalizations, a necessity for multiple, highly sophisticated medical procedures and specialists from numerous fields of medicine including infectious disease, oncology, hematology, and pharmacology, to name a few. Often these specialists must be involved to control raging infection and unbelievable complications. The post hospital care is similarly complex. As the illness progresses, debilitation is the rule rather than the exception, and unemployment is usual.

Complications of the central nervous system (CNS) can result in more psychological stress and further behavioral change. These complications may even impair one's ability to carry out daily routines, to care for oneself, and more importantly, to cope with the devastating illness.

When we refer to the neuropsychiatric complications of the disease, we are referring primarily to central nervous system infections; subacute encephalitis is the old term for what is now called AIDS encephalopathy. The psychiatric complications are primarily depression, anxiety, delirium, and dementia. In a series of 50 patients with AIDS at Memorial Sloan-Kettering Cancer Center who developed CNS infections, more than half of these patients had neurologic complications expressed as some form of subacute encephalitis.[1] It is believed that the HTLV-III virus is implicated here, accounting for most of the cases. Thirty-one percent of patients in this series have an abnormal neurological examination in general. At autopsy, however, CNS involvement was noted in 78% of those autopsied. Thus, nervous system involvement was present without a positive neurologic examination. More recent work has shown the HTLV-III virus to have a high affinity for nervous tissue.[2]

In the early stages of the infection, central nervous system complications are quite indistinguishable from depression. I have been called to see patients for what appears to be depression; later, we determined that their symptoms were caused by a central nervous system infection. The symptoms are quite indistinguishable. Patients experience headaches and depressed mood. They have difficulty concentrating, which progresses; the clarity and rapidity of thinking is slowed. They experience a loss of libido, and a loss of interest in both work and social involvement. There is diminished quality and quantity of work; performance is seriously impaired over time. There is a slow withdrawal from social contacts. I think it is important to keep these symptoms in mind when we see an AIDS patient who appears depressed.

Later, as the CNS infection progresses, a delirium can be seen with confusion, disorientation, memory loss, agitated behavior, and even coma. Some patients have had seizures and have developed dementia and other central nervous system illnesses.

On the psychiatry service between January 1982 and July 1983, we saw 23 AIDS patients, about 15% of the total AIDS cases seen at Memorial Sloan-Kettering Hospital. We were called to see these patients for the following reasons: most of the patients were depressed and we were called in to help manage their depression; three patients expressed a desire to die and planned to do so by taking their own lives; seven patients exhibited some form of abnormal social behavior. We used the Diagnostic and Statistical Manual of Mental Disorders of the American Psychiatric Association[3] as a diagnostic tool. We saw psychiatric problems in 17 of our 23 patients related directly to their diagnosis of AIDS. Thirteen patients showed some form of an reactive adjustment disorder resulting from abnormal emotional response to the illness; three patients had organic mental disorders; and one patient exhibited a brief reactive psychosis. Five patients had preexisting psychiatric problems before they were diagnosed with AIDS.

In consulting with these patients, a constellation of symptoms is very obvious to the observer. Ninety-one percent exhibited some feelings of isolation; depressed mood was very common as well (78%); low self-esteem and suicidal thoughts were often present. Suicidal thoughts occurred in some of the patients immediately after they received the diagnosis. As we worked with these patients, however, the desire to die waned, especially as they became more comfortable and started mobilizing to obtain health care. Interestingly enough, guilt was not common among all the consultation samples.

In this group of 23 patients, neurological complications were eventually present in 14. We followed the patients through the course of their illness. When these patients died, of those autopsied, eight had positive neurological findings; it is very possible that what was diagnosed as depression and adjustment disorders with depressed mood may have actually been the beginnings of central nervous system infection. Patients who are depressed may very well have neurological involvement; this is a critical perspective to keep in mind when treating AIDS patients.

With respect to psychiatric treatment, psychotherapy, of a crisis intervention nature, was effective in a number of our patients. We used psychotropic medications for a number of others. Low dose antidepressants helped to make some people much more comfortable; we used major tranquilizers for patients who exhibited a delirium.

Also, we found social service referrals to be very useful in our intervention. The services of the Gay Men's Health Crisis in New York City was used quite often. In many situations, their input was critical in assisting the patient to cope with the illness.

Mental Health Needs of People with AIDS

Marshall Forstein, M.D.
Instructor in Psychiatry, Harvard Medical School
Staff Psychiatrist, The Cambridge City Hospital
Medical Director, The Gay and Lesbian
Counseling Service

The mental health issues that are being raised at this time are not simply how to deal with people with AIDS and the psychiatric implications of a patient having a deadly disease. The mental health implications of the development of the ELISA test for HTLV-III screening are becoming apparent on a relatively frequent basis. Every person in America will be affected by this epidemic.

The most apparent need for mental health services exists in those people who have AIDS. There is a significant body of scientific literature about young, terminally ill people and how they cope with it. One problem with the mental health of patients with AIDS is that they are not always sick, as such. Patients are subjected to a roller coaster, fluctuating illness that will instill hope through wellness, then serious depression when illness becomes apparent. The nature of the mental health needs vary from moment to moment. In the people trained to deal with these needs, an interface seems to exist between the medical aspects and the psychological and psychosocial aspects of the disease. It is no longer possible for nonmedically trained people to avoid dealing with this illness; people, both medical and nonmedical, are talking constantly about the psychological and medical needs of people with AIDS. When a crisis intervention worker gets a call from someone with AIDS who is depressed or suicidal, the worker should begin to think about the possibilities of an organic etiology that needs immediate attention due to the nature of the underlying immune deficiency. It requires a certain amount of skill and agility for social scientists to develop this interface with medicine, but it is essential that it be done. The physical and mental health needs of the patient require social and medical practitioners to work closely together.

My experience with this disease relates primarily to working with people who have the psychiatric manifestations of AIDS, once they have been discharged from the hospital. This is not only a disease affecting gay men. People who are IV drug abusers, or patients who suffer from hemophilia all have mental health needs, especially in light of their social environment. People at risk need to understand their relationship to society. It is hard to refute the proposition that gay men, as a group, have been historically and are, at present, an oppressed minority group. A patient with AIDS suffers oppression from white and black America; hemophiliacs, who once looked to the advances of science as life-giving, now have the perspective that some of these advances are lifethreatening.

We have only begun to understand the implications of the disease on the mental and social health of these groups.

Our understanding of the mental health of people with AIDS or AIDS-related complex is woefully inadequate. These people are walking around feeling very much like time bombs, not knowing who among them will develop AIDS. The data suggest that anywhere from 4% to 19% of these people who are diagnosed with HTLV-III antibody positive may, at some point in the future, develop AIDS. In my experience, some people with AIDS have fared better, psychologically, than some people with AIDS-related complex (ARC) who had a much more fluctuating physical course. This latter group has a very difficult time dealing with existing without a sense of what will happen to them. A number of patients with AIDS have expressed to me some relief at having a clear diagnosis, with a sense of mission, of purpose, a sense of how they can take control of their lives. It appears to be more difficult when you are walking around in a field of land mines and you do not know where you are stepping, what will happen, when it will happen, or whether you will be the next one to get hit. Some people in this group experience a wide range of psychiatric problems, including acute anxiety, beginning even before diagnosis, and a very high incidence of suicidal thinking and ideation. In my experience, there seems to be initially an acute period of anxiety, with some leveling off with time as support systems and contact with mental health providers experienced with the disease increases. In a conceptual sense, people never quite return to the previous level of relative personal calm. Events in their lives that previously may have been handled quite well suddenly become major precipitants of new anxieties. I believe it is due to this chronic uncertainty and lack of control over their own lives. For example, if someone loses an apartment, he otherwise might have said, "Well, I'll find another place to live." With the addition of this minor irritant in light of the disease-related stress, it may become a tremendous precipitant to new anxiety, with a new lowering of self-esteem. These people tend to have serious problems coping with otherwise normal human experiences.

It is especially important, as we learn more about central nervous system involvement in AIDS, that mental changes, behavioral changes, and attitudinal changes be evaluated in light of the possible organic basis for the behavior. It becomes an imperative that an organic etiology be considered in people who are HTLV-III positive and particularly in people who are diagnosed as having ARC. While we still cannot adequately treat the underlying immune deficiency, we do know that a sensorium change due to a nonviral etiology, such as a toxoplasmosis infection, can be treated, to some extent, with our present armamentarium. It is imperative then that we see the mental health needs of the patient in light of the possible organic basis for the psychiatric illness.

We are beginning to see considerable societal stress in an ever-widening circle of people, regardless of whether the person is rationally at risk. At the alternative

HTLV-III testing site in Massachusetts, people are asking questions such as "I had an anonymous sexual encounter 12 years ago, nothing since, and I am afraid I have been infected." Rationally, we may be able to say there is very, very little risk of being exposed, but the fear of being exposed is the mental health issue. Also, we have people who are not themselves exposed or at high risk but who are so afraid of being around people that are at high risk that we begin to understand the statements of people like Jerry Falwell and some local senators here in Massachusetts who would quarantine all people at risk. Regardless of whether people are in high risk groups, we have to understand that their own anxiety about the uncertainty of the illness engenders all sorts of fears and paranoia. I have received phone calls from people wanting to know which restaurants should be avoided due to a higher preponderance of gay patrons or gay waiters. Notwithstanding the irrational nature of these perspectives, the people expressing the fears are afraid; I am afraid that we will see more of this in the future.

The mental health needs of people at risk need to be tailored again to the specific kinds of problems that are imagined by these people. When a married man who has had an occasional, extramarital sexual encounter calls, he cannot be told that he is not at risk. One has to have a very comprehensive understanding of the nature of the dual life he is leading, the nature of the oppression that he feels, the nature of the denial of guilt among other things. These issues cannot be alleviated by administering the HTLV-III antibody test. How people such as this use mental health services depends on the societal attitude about the need for those mental health services. Funding for mental health services has never been a priority in our society. When we have people with longstanding schizophrenic or manic-depressive illnesses living on the streets because we do not make it a priority to house these people, it is not hard to imagine what is in store for the large numbers of HTLV-III positive individuals.

When a health care practitioner is confronted with a person who has AIDS, someone who imagines himself or herself at risk, or the sexual partner of someone who is HTLV-III positive, it is important that these practitioners be well-trained and educated about the mental aspects of the disease process. It should not be assumed that people adequately trained in other mental health issues will be qualified to deal with some of these issues. It is important to determine and address the educational needs of mental health professionals. It will become increasingly important to pay attention to education from the beginning of professional training so that an understanding of the psychological needs of people at risk may be enhanced. For many people with AIDS, the medical provider serves a very real psychological function. The patient becomes psychologically dependent on their caregiver; often, it is the only family for people who have been otherwise abandoned or left without a social support structure. We need to reinforce to these caregivers that medical people cannot only be technicians. They must understand that as a human being talking to another human being, they have a direct responsibility to pay attention to the fact that there is a person on the other side of that illness. It is not clear that medical training alone can develop this sense of responsibility in a health care provider. Usually, this caring is brought to medical or nursing school with the person. These patients need to have a sense of belonging, a sense that someone values them, that someone supports their sense of self. The patients are vulnerable to thinking there is something inherently wrong with them.

When a society says homosexual men, by virtue of their sexual practices, are guilty of a crime, it is important to realize that this perspective has a direct and significant impact on the sense of oneself, on the capacity to cope, and on a feeling of belonging to the world. A person's mental health is directly correlated with the social acclaim or disclaim that people are confronted with or exposed to. When people lose their jobs or are financially unable to support themselves, then the incidence of mental disease increases. Why does a patient who is diagnosed as having AIDS want to die? Perhaps this emotional reaction stems from his knowledge about his role as an outcast, as someone who doesn't belong and is not valued as a human being. As a learning exercise, consider your thoughts about a two-year-old child you see toddling down the street. I do not know anyone who intrinsically hates a two-year-old child; one could get angry with him on occasion, but it does not rise to a level of disgust or hatred, even in a stranger's two-year-old. As these two-year-old children age, some of them become 25-year-old gay men or IV drug abusers. The early intrinsic warmth for a two-year-old sometimes changes to an evil, distant, cold, perhaps hating feeling for a 25-year-old. What happened? Why do we suddenly go from loving to hating the person? This is one issue we have to deal with when we address mental health issues, primarily because the mental health of an individual is directly related to the mental health of our whole society. At some point, all of us deal with the notion of death and dying. None of us are spared. AIDS victims deal with this before they are supposed to and in light of a tremendous amount of pressure that was never anticipated. Mental health professionals need to creatively address their needs. It can only be done, in my opinion, by integrating their mental and physical health care needs through social policy change and relevant legislative action.

To Have Without Holding:
Memories of Life with a Person with AIDS

Joseph Interrante, Ph.D.
Lecturer, Harvard University
Member and Former Chair of Education,
AIDS Action Committee in Boston

Our love and hate for the body remain inaccessible to and unreconciled with each other so long as the full recognition of our mortality that would bring them together remains beyond our emotional strength. And the pooled inventiveness and striving which constitute our species' self-creation have been from the outset contaminated . . . by these unreconciled feelings for the flesh: the basic way of life that distinguishes us from other creatures is distorted . . . by this refusal to face death.[4]

The fear of death hovers over all physician–patient encounters and not only over those with dying patients. . . . Doctors have an intriguing love–hate relationship with death: It is both their ally and their enemy. In trying to defeat death, physicians are death's adversaries. When physicians borrow the power engendered by patients' fear of death for purposes of control, death is their ally. . . . Physicians struggle against and embrace of death can cast a dark shadow over another covert struggle between physicians and patients: how life is to be lived. Life, including the life of an illness, can be lived in myriads of ways, and not only according to the views of physicians. . . . [But] doctors view death as a personal defeat rather than an eventual inevitability to which they, like their patients, must submit.[5]

I am the life-partner of a gay man who died from AIDS in October, 1983. Our experience during the seven months that followed Paul DiAngelo's diagnosis in March, 1983 was shaped by our social backgrounds, the history of our relationship, the particular configurations of Paul's illness, and the specific place in the history of AIDS in which our experience occurred. I recount this experience below because many aspects of it are instructive about the impact of AIDS. A great deal of the experience was not pleasant.

Both of us were white, professional men in our early thirties who had been together for five and a half years. Paul and I had settled into a relationship with its own rituals and traditions, with a network of friends tied to us as a couple or to one of us as individuals, and with an accumulation of trust and mutual dependence that facilitated rather easily the reordering of our lives around Paul's illness. The merging of financial resources and the drawing up of legal protections, for example, raised no questions about the durability of our relationship, questions which might have occurred had our relationship been younger.[6] At the same time, the fact that Paul was one of the first 14 confirmed cases of AIDS in

Boston, at a time when AIDS was still a foreign experience to most people inside and outside the Boston gay community, also colored our life. Paul's work, and through him, my work with the AIDS Action Committee as media "representatives" of the AIDS experience forced us consciously to think about and to articulate our changing perspectives on life with AIDS. This intensified our processes of self-reflection and evaluation and also helped to alleviate some of the isolation which characterized living with AIDS in Boston in 1983.

AIDS fundamentally restructured the rhythms and routines of our life together. My memories of those seven months are marked by the milestones in Paul's illness: the flu that would not go away in late February; the diagnosis of Kaposi's sarcoma and interstitial pneumonitis in March; the increasing fatigue and diarrhea in April; the visits to Paul's health center for intravenous treatments for his dehydration in early May; his admission to the hospital in late May, and the diagnosis of cryptospirosis a few days later; his inability to absorb nutrition and the resultant IV feeding in June; the spreading cancer and recurrence of pneumonia in July; the surgery to implant a Hickman catheter in his chest in August; his return home later that month; the steady decline in weight and strength and the hallucinations in September; and, finally, his death in October.

Daily life became ordered by the demands of health care. We took trips by taxi to his health center and social service agencies in March, April, and May. I visited him daily at the hospital in June, July, and August. After he returned home, I scheduled AIDS Action Committee support service volunteers and friends to care for him while I was at work. I maintained the nightly routines of home health care and housework in September and October. The experience was frequently an exhausting one of days, nights, weeks, months of turning on and off the IVAC pump, of ordering and storing medical supplies, of fetching this and taking away that. Errands of sorrow and joy, errands of mercy, errands of hopeful and despairing love.[7] Within those rhythms and routines, we carved out time for us alone. A time to recount and share the events of the day, a time to weigh the possibilities and probabilities of illness and recovery, a time to maintain and sustain a life, and gradually a time to create a death of our own.

Our effort to create a life and death of our own was not without opposition, especially during Paul's three months in the hospital. Numerous instances, some of which Paul recorded in his journals and others witnessed by me, exemplified what Katz calls "the silent world of doctor and patient"—an unwillingness or inability to involve Paul in discussion and decisionmaking about how his illness was to be lived. On the other hand, I witnessed a dramatic change in the manner of his primary physician who did learn to listen, to discuss, and eventually to accept and support Paul's wishes about his death. Perhaps as an oncologist this doctor was more used to death. But the experience of someone his own age dying, whom he could not save, was I believe less familiar, and it certainly took its emotional toll. I have seen this pattern of intense physician involvement, acceptance, and acquiescence become more common in the last two years. In our focus on medical research, however, this development has been overlooked, despite or perhaps because of its exemplary potential for breaking through the silence which has customarily governed the theory and practice of doctor–patient relations.

As Paul slowly realized and came to terms with the probability of his death, he began to settle what he called the "unfinished business" in his life, to complete his relationships with parents, sister, former lovers, and friends, and to complete our relationship. His physical decline was accompanied by psychological and emotional growth. In that sense, AIDS condensed and compressed into months the decades of normal living.

Paul's life and our relationship together had been based upon openness and communication. AIDS infused our interactions with intensity and urgency, particularly on my behalf. Because of the trust and honesty in our relationship which was confirmed in the face of this crisis, Paul allowed himself to rely physically and emotionally upon me. He let himself go in unique ways with me. With friends and with kin he struggled to maintain his self-reliance, to struggle out of bed (until he could no longer lift himself) into the bathroom—an event which took place at least 20 times a day. With me, he would allow himself to be lifted and carried, to have his food cut up and to be fed to him, to be washed like an infant. With me, he would explore the conflicting emotions raised by his increasing physical dependence—his hopes for recovery, his anger at the illness, his disappointment over reversals and relapses. Together we worked through his sense of powerlessness, his feelings of resignation, his gradual acceptance of death, or rather, I should say "our" feelings. I was drawn into Paul's illness which not only ordered my own life but tempered my emotional status. His needs became my needs; his hopes and disappointments, mine. When asked by friends, "How are you doing?" I would often reply with an account of Paul's current condition, his psychological state, and my feelings about him. In fact, I think at times that my disappointment over relapses, my anger at callous treatment by friends, was more intense than his. I did not have the physical symptoms to contend with in an immediate way, but I watched him struggle with his illness and saw how events and people hurt him. I could not eliminate the symptoms or the pain; I could only help him persevere.

The closest model with which to compare my experience during those seven months of life with Paul is the experience of mothering. My mother brought this home to me when she said after being told of Paul's death, "The hardest thing in the world to bear is the death of a child or a mate." By this analogy I mean the cluster of activities, characteristics, and emotions associated with the social role of motherhood.[8] Whether performed by women or by men, mothering and its analogue within the health care system, nursing, involves the intimate physical care of another being, the provision of unconditional caring and love, the subordination of self to others, and an investment in separation. Indeed, as Paul's condition worsened and his body became hypersensitized to pain, our ability to use touching to express love narrowed. An arm draped lightly over his chest while we slept eventually created too much pressure so that we learned to sleep together without touching. A hug caused pain, not pleasure, so that we restricted ourselves to his resting his hand over mine or my lightly caressing his cheek with my forefinger. As his body became bloated from inactivity, his speech slurred from medication, his talking painful because breathing was painful, we learned to communicate love through a glance. As these forms of erotic touch disappeared, my consciousness of the love-infusing acts of physical care was heightened.

Many of my memories during those seven months are visceral. Memories of the body associated with the touch of intimate physical care, shampooing his hair, washing his back, shaving his face in the hospital. At home, I remember changing the bandages around his Hickman catheter, moving him on the bed, lifting him out of bed and onto the portable toilet, cleaning and changing him when he became incontinent, feeding him crushed frozen juices. Watching the gay man carry his lover upstairs in Lanford Wilson's *Fifth of July* triggers a semantic response in me that is inadequately conveyed in words. It is a response grounded in the memories of physical care, the memories of watching a man's capacities for physical self-reliance regress to those of a one-year-old child; memories of a vibrant and young man's life trapped in the body of a feeble old man. It is a response rooted in my learning to accept his death, learning to thwart the reflexes of grab and touch, learning to love and let go, learning to have and not to hold.[9] This is Paul's legacy to me as I reinvest in the various forms of gay singlehood, build new relationships with old friends as well as new ones, and reenter a community more conscious of and intimately involved with AIDS. Through Paul's willingness to draw me into his illness, he taught me to face death. By facing and becoming part of his death, I have confronted my own love and hate for the body, and for the limits and mortality of my own existence. That sense of mortality, of judicious responsibility for myself and for others has become a part of me. Like wearing a ring or a pair of eyeglasses, I have grown used to it, and I will never forget it.[10] Beyond the partially successful efforts to articulate this experience through language, my body will remember it and will never forget it because I don't want to forget.

Social Impact on Dating in the Gay Community

David McWhirter, M.D.
Assistant Clinical Professor of Psychiatry
University of California at San Diego School of Medicine
Co-Director, Clinical Institute for
Human Relationships, San Diego

One of the powerful things about being a physician, a psychotherapist, or other health caregiver is the manner that patients trust you because of your position and your caring attitude. Physician–patient relationships develop very quickly. I want to discuss one such relationship.

Ben was 34-years old when he came to see me in the fall of 1980. He was a gorgeous, young, gay man who was terribly depressed, self-effacing, self-negative, and having a lot of difficulty with his own internalized homophobia. He had two master's degrees and a good job, but was not functioning very well on that job. He was seeking assistance from me in getting his life straightened out. He did remarkably well in therapy, and by the summer of 1981, he had entered into a stable relationship with a man, had made arrangements for a new job, and was moving along in the whole process of becoming a full, functioning member of society. He left my care in March, 1982. He had been ill for the previous three weeks; he did not know what was the matter and looked very sick. He had seen a local physician who knew very little about AIDS. He was then seen by a skilled physician. Ten days later, he died from a pneumocystis carinii infection. What happens to us as health care providers when a patient dies like my patient did? Do we somehow manage to "buck up" and move on to take care of the next patient? I have treated 37 patients with AIDS; 17 of them are already dead. I have not yet learned to cope with the losses of patients who are young and healthy.

One of the ways in which I have attempted to assist patients in this epidemic is by lecturing in various communities. I can determine almost immediately whether AIDS is an issue in the area I am lecturing. If there are a few cases of AIDS and they are not concerned about AIDS in the community, the reactions to my discussions are not very well developed. As soon as I meet some people in that community who know men who have AIDS or have friends in other places who have AIDS, I see a different set of reactions. Thus, public perception of the illness and the public health approach to this disease varies. It has a lot to do with people's awareness of those who are ill and having a contact with those who have contracted this disease. In many places, I think, we are seeing sex as usual and I am not certain why it is still happening. Perhaps people are reacting to AIDS-related deaths in the same way thousands react to automobile accidents each year. Many people still drive while intoxicated. The process of denial appears to appears to be operating in a similar manner in gay people's attitudes about sexual exclusivity and relationships.

Drew Madison (my life-partner for the last 14 years) and I began a research project in 1974 to evaluate gay male relationships over a period of five years, from 1975 to 1979. We interviewed 156 couples, many of them in depth over several years' time. We had some longitudinal quality to this study. The couples were together from one year to 37½ years, with over 75% of the men together for over five years. None of the men together over five years, in the our original sample, had an ongoing expectation of sexual exclusivity in their relationships; namely, they had some outside sexual contacts after the fifth year of the relationship. There were many sexual encounters in the first few years of relationships, especially in those people who had agreements about such sexual activity. In the last year, we have reinterviewed 25 of the original 156 couples. Of these 25 couples, all of them have reduced their outside sexual risk. Eighteen couples have reported a return to early relationship expectations of sexual exclusivity. Thus, there appears to have been a large shift back to sexual exclusivity. Every person interviewed has reported serious concerns and anxiety about AIDS.

We have started a new project this year where we are interviewing couples who have been together for over 20 years. Of 22 couples, 14 couples had not had sexual contact with each other for anywhere from one year to 11 years. Interestingly enough, in the couples interviewed that were together for more than 20 years, if they previously had not been having sexual contact with each other, there appears to be a reawakening or a new investment in some kind of sexual contact with each other. I am not certain why, but it may stem from an interest in reducing the risk of transmitting AIDS from other sexual partners to their life-partner.

As you are all aware, a recent study involved gay men who were presented with all available information about HTLV-III antibody testing.[11] The men were told that the only value to the antibody testing was to screen for contaminated blood. A questionnaire to these individuals was handed out; in response, 70% of the group still reported that they would take the test because they wanted to find out the result of their HTLV-III antibody test. I think this result is critical to maintain the availability of the blood supply, and is one of the major reasons why setting up alternate test sites has become such an important program. Another study in San Diego yielded similar results.[12]

I think that there has been a great shift in the gay male community at the present time. More gay men appear to be recognizing that it would be easier if they were in relationships. Gay men appear to be looking for partners with a great deal more anxiety and more effort than they have before and, as a consequence, this has become a very central theme. In the presence of this anxiety, it is even more difficult to get a partner. Everyone is so frightened at what the outcome of a sexual encounter may be.

Another change in the behavior of gay men in the process of coupling is that they are going back to doing a lot of dating. Many of my patients are dating for months before they have a sexual encounter with the man they have been pursuing. It is somewhat adolescent in that the couples are entertaining each other but abstaining from sex.

In our original sample of couples, somewhere near 60% of them had sex with each other before they knew each other's names. So there is a definite real change over the past decade in the process of coupling, which I attribute to the AIDS epidemic. We are just beginning to understand the behavioral changes that public perception of this disease is causing.

Social Support Services: AIDS Action Committees

Lawrence Kessler
Coordinator, AIDS Action Committee, Boston
Member, Mayor's Task Force on AIDS

It was very apparent early in 1982 that the AIDS epidemic in the gay community was exceedingly serious. It was about that time that the Gay Men's Health Crisis in New York, the Kaposi's Sarcoma Foundation in San Francisco and Houston, and the AIDS Action Committee in Boston began to meet to try to define the extent of the crisis and some possible approaches to addressing the key issues. Basically, we had to do something if we expected those people who had AIDS or anxiety about AIDS to get help. By 1983, there were 45 groups around the country, providing support and advocacy for patients and their families, lovers, and friends. The groups made certain that patients got what they needed when they were in the hospital and later, if they were discharged from the hospital, that they were treated like people. Educational needs about the disease AIDS were met. The patients were told of their legal rights. Other educational issues included assisting the families to adjust to the diagnosis, to deal with the implication of being gay, and to understand what AIDS was and how it was spread. Also, there was a need to educate civic leaders and concerned public health departments. In essence, it was the gay community in those 45 cities and later, around the world, that began to raise money, consciousness, and a sense of responsibility so that those people who had AIDS could get what they needed.

The AIDS Action Committee is a volunteer agency, with a staff of five, approximately 150 to 175 volunteers, and a budget of $300,000. One-third of that amount has been raised in the community through fundraisers, collections at bars, and memorial donations made in honor of those who died. Another third comes from the City of Boston. The last third comes from a combination of state funds and either research grants or direct funding for hotline and hotline staff. Our anticipated budget for next year is $500,000; it will include additional staff, more volunteers, social workers, and health coordinators. We receive $200,000 in in-kind services from volunteers in Boston. In New York, the Gay Men's Health Crisis has received over 200,000 hours of volunteer time, and, if valued by in-kind contributions, a several million dollar social service agency is functioning.

The Action Committee is managed by a steering committee made up of 10 subcommittees. Each subcommittee elects a chair, and that chairperson is appointed to the steering committee. The staff has a mandate, a job description, and a mission that is developed by the steering committee to meet the needs at hand.

In Boston, the Action Committee has worked closely with public officials. There has been a level of trust between the AIDS Action Committee, its staff, the Committee's volunteer members and the public health officials. It does not necessarily mean that we have always agreed on the proper approach, but rather that we have had a sense of community and purpose. We have managed to overcome the personal and political ego so that we can provide better services to people with AIDS. Collaboration between cities, states, and the federal government is essential. While the government has the money that we need, we have a storehouse of talent, expertise, and knowledge about AIDS. Cooperation is essential, especially because 75% of the AIDS cases in Massachusetts involve gay or bisexual people. Thus, in such a populous state, the government has a vested interest in ensuring the health of the populace, that people with AIDS are served at all levels, whether it be in the hospital, mental health centers, or at home.

Whatever the local group may be called, I suggest that you will find that the work that you are doing—whether it be in the lab, on the wards, or in your private practices—will be greatly enhanced by the talent and abilities of the kinds of people who have joined these committees.

Another issue that is startling is the current cost of caring for people with AIDS. For the 9,500 patients who have AIDS, the health care costs alone exceed $1 billion; the productivity costs exceeds $4 billion over the course of what would normally be the rest of these patients' lives. This does not include the loss of tax dollars to the government. Next year, when we add another 9,500 patients, we are going to repeat that process. Is it sensible to invest $85 million in AIDS research when we are expending $1 billion in health care (which does not cure the disease) for the current 9,500 patients who have the disease? We should allocate another $85 million to address the issues relating to heterosexual transmission cofactors, and another $85 million for patient care, support, housing, and mental health services. Perhaps then we might be able to say that we are doing an adequate job of addressing the AIDS issue. The whole question of research is a difficult one because of the issues of confidentiality and informed consent, in addition to the issue of funding programs solely at the federal level or at the NIH. There is precedent for research funds to funnel down to teaching hospitals, to clinics, and to labs all across the country. We may not find the cure or the breakthrough at the local level. Then again we may, in the middle of the night, discover an important key somewhere in a nongovernment lab.

In the future, I hope that the manner in which the committees have responded to this crisis will have given rise to the development of a working model for collaboration between the medical world and the community. This model could be useful unless a large manpower need arises for education, caring, and mobilization of community reserves.

Question

(Steve Glicken, Tufts University): Please comment on any "burn-out" or emotional problems which have developed in people who are working as members of the committees.

Answer

Burn-out is a serious problem for volunteers. To our credit, however, we have turned a tremendous amount of pressure and stress in working with people with AIDS into self-support networks. For example, nurses involved in caring for AIDS patients are establishing support groups to help nurses to address their feelings. Sometimes we recommend rotating staff through the most difficult positions to give people a chance to recover and to set limits.

Early in the epidemic, I was seeing people with AIDS or ARC, and I went through periods when I had to step back from the on-site contacts. I was contributing but acknowledged that I could only cope with a certain amount of the stress until I needed a break. Where can the caretakers seek support for needs? This is an area that needs a great deal more exploration. The frustration exists at every level. Everybody involved with this problem at some level needs other people to work with, to respond to their emotional needs to be able to honestly say, "I've had enough today, I need to go home; don't call me." As our numbers increase, we will have increasing numbers of people who are going to be asked to deal with AIDS, ARC, and HTLV-III positivity. What about the person in the small community mental health center who may be the only person dealing with these issues? We need to pay attention to his needs for support and ongoing education. The Committee has tried to offer some support to the caretakers, through positive feedback and critical evaluations, especially if people are not doing what they need to do. But sometimes we even use symbols. We have sent baskets of flowers to eight or nine providers for their help, saying, "It's a nice time of the year to thank you for all the things you've been doing for people with AIDS and we're appreciative of it, and we hope to continue to work with you through the year." We have also done that with nurses, particularly after a long, gruesome or involved stay on a particular floor where everyone was involved. We tried to acknowledge their commitment through a simple but heartfelt gift, such as flowers. We believe it is important for the caregivers because this disease takes its toll on everyone, with no exceptions.

Comment

(John Mazzullo, M.D., Tufts University School of Medicine): As many people have suggested, in the history of medicine there have been very few instances where an illness such as AIDS has had such incredible psychosocial impact. My own experience with this illness as a physician (and a gay physician) was somewhat theoretical until 1981. I did not have much personal or professional experience with the disease (nor did anyone else) until I met a patient, Bill, at the Medical Center who was diagnosed as having AIDS. Bill became a personal friend of mine and, when Bill was discharged, we kept in occasional contact with each other. One day, I saw Bill at my health club. I was very relieved to see that Bill was not in the hospital and was functioning in society again. It became very clear to me that I had to get some sense of this illness when I turned the corner at the health club to go into the hot tub, and there was Bill sitting in the hot tub. I had to make a decision at that moment—a very personal, very difficult decision—as to whether I would turn around and leave my buddy, my friend, or whether I was going to take the acceptable risk of getting into the hot tub with him. Let me assure you that I did a lot of reading in the medical texts later that night about chlorine and the alternation of viruses because I was somewhat frightened. To have turned away from him would have been something I could not have done. Everyone has his or her own story about this illness and how it has become real and palpable, and not just a story of viruses and T-lymphocytes.

Lastly, the mental health impact of this illness is staggering and, from my perspective, the response of government has been incredibly slow in freeing up funds for mental health counseling. Many of our discussions relate only to hospitalized AIDS patients; the submerged part of the iceberg is the "well" patient who goes through serious depressive cycles, such as Bill.

Unfortunately, there is some evidence for the proposition that some of the opportunistic infections affect central nervous system processes, and newer data show that the AIDS retrovirus affects neurological tissue. The fact that the disease itself can affect psychologic and neurologic function raises serious legal questions of competency and other confounding issues.

References

1. Snider, W.D., D.M. Simpson, S. Nielson, et al. 1983. Neurological complications of acquired immune deficiency syndrome: analysis of 50 patients. *Annals of Neurology* 14(4):403–418.
2. Epstein, L.G., D.C. Gajducek, R.W. Price, et al. 1985. HTLV-III infection encephalopathy. *Science* 227:177–182.
3. American Psychiatric Association. 1980. *Diagnostic and Statistical Manual of Mental Disorders.* 3rd edition. Washington, DC: American Psychiatric Press.
4. Dinnerstein, Dorothy. 1976. *The mermaid and the minotaur: sexual arrangements and human malaise.* New York: Harper and Row.
5. Katz, Jay. 1984. *The silent world of doctor and patient.* New York: Free Press.
6. See, for example, David McWhirter and Andrew Mattison. 1984. *The male couple: how relationships develop.* Englewood Cliffs, NJ: Prentice-Hall.
7. The phrases are adapted from Joseph Hansen. 1973. *Death Claims.* New York: Harper and Row.
8. On mothering, see Dinnerstein, *Mermaid and minotaur;* Nancy Chodorow. 1978. The reproduction of mothering: psychoanalysis and the sociology of gender. Berkeley: University of California Press; Diane Ehrensaft. 1980. When women and men mother. *Socialist Review* no. 49:37–73.
9. The phrases come from a poem by Marge Piercy, "To Have Without Holding."
10. The analogy comes from Harvey Fierstein, *Torch Song Trilogy,* "Women and Children First!", scene 4.
11. Moran, Steve. 1985. Report to the Advisory Task Force to California Legislature on AIDS, February.
12. McKusick, Leon. 1985. Report to the Advisory Task Force to California Legislature on AIDS, February.

PART VI
HTLV-III Screening and the Blood Supply

Public Health Policies and Concerns

Kenneth Mayer, M.D.
Assistant Professor of Medicine, Brown University
Chief, Division of Infectious Diseases,
Memorial Hospital, Pawtucket, Rhode Island
Research Director, Fenway Community Health Center

I have encountered a variety of ironies and difficulties with the current state of knowledge regarding HTLV-III screening and the ELISA test. At the onset of the AIDS epidemic, and before the HTLV-III screening test was available, I was confronted by worried patients who articulated physical and emotional distress. Some of these patients had minimal symptomatology but major concerns; others met the criteria established by the CDC for AIDS. Many patients wanted a definitive test. At that time, many wanted to have T-lymphocyte helper–suppressor ratio tests performed. I explained to each client that various processes such as intercurrent viral infections could influence the result of the test.

Later, once the ELISA test became available, it was ironic that many people subsequently did not want to have the test performed. There has been a tendency for certain individuals in the highest risk groups who are already ostracized by society to want to bury the messenger bearing the bad news. The alienation of gay men and IV drug users regarding the ELISA test has been abetted by the "Science by Press Conference" approach of Secretary Heckler and colleagues, and the rapid overinterpretation of both test results and their clinical significance. Although the etiologic agent of AIDS is the retrovirus, HTLV-III/LAV, other cofactors may contribute significantly to the pathogenesis of AIDS. There may be other factors that determine which individuals exposed to the virus become infected or whether infected individuals progress to clinical illness. However, at this time we are not certain what these cofactors are. Exposures to other viruses such as cytomegalovirus and Epstein-Barr virus, drugs such as volatile nitrites, and genetic factors have been postulated as modulators of HTLV-III infection. But why some exposed persons stay well for years and others rapidly get sick remains unclear. Thus, there are good reasons to question the diagnostic utility of the test since it does not confer perfect information. In Chicago, for example, there is a brochure that questions the meaning of the results of the antibody test by saying "Flip a coin." Because some studies of seropositivity in the gay community averaged approximately 50% in Chicago, the drafters of the brochure suggest that if one flips a coin one could determine, just as well as the test would, whether one has an increased risk for the disease. However, further studies of the ELISA test indicate that in AIDS risk groups, the predictive value of a positive test is high, so the problem is one of clinical interpretation. Does knowing that one has a 6% chance of developing AIDS over six years help in coping with life stresses and behavioral change? Would all persons who knew they were HTLV-III antibody positive only perform safe sex or would a negative result lead to continuation of unsafe practices?

If we look at hepatitis B screening as an analogy, we find a different situation. In gay communities where hepatitis B exposure is frequent, the prevalence of markers to hepatitis B antibody may be as high as 50% with a minority of persons giving a history of clinical illness. We routinely test for the presence of hepatitis B. We routinely brand persons as carriers of hepatitis virus and often discover the presence of chronic liver disease. One important distinction between hepatitis B screening and HTLV-III testing at the present time is that a vaccine is available for the former virus but not the latter. When we test people we often can only give individuals ambiguous answers; other times, we may have more concrete solutions. Persons with hepatitis B serologic markers are a heterogeneous group. Some of those individuals may be determined to be core antibody positive (Hb$_c$Ab) or have persistence of the surface antigen (Hb$_s$Ag). Those individuals may be chronic carriers requiring special precautions but have varying expression of the illness. Subsequent tests will not tell us which persons will become debilitated by hepatitis for the balance of their lives with cirrhosis of the liver or hepatocellular carcinoma (liver cancer) or whether they will stay well. Health providers can use the test results to counsel clients so as to protect uninfected persons.

The HTLV-III virus diagnostic tests are at an early stage of development. We expect to see HTLV-III antigen tests, easier methods of viral isolation, and improved "second generation" antibody tests soon. Thus, an informed decision must be made by both the clinician and patient as to whether to use the currently available HTLV-III ELISA test. Some people simplistically urge testing everyone at risk now; others scorn this possibility. A nonrhetorical consensus remains to be achieved.

Last spring, Dr. Donald Francis, a virologist at the CDC, suggested that all homosexually active males should be tested immediately so that seropositive people could have sexual contact with other seropositive people and seronegatives could have sexual contact with seronegatives. However, an HTLV-III antibody negative yet viral culture positive state exists. Encouraging people who are seronegative to meet other seronegative people is understandable, but fails to appreciate the biology—some people may have the virus in their bodies but have not had sufficient time to mount an antibody response detectable by the commercially available ELISA tests, while others may never make antibodies after certain viral exposures, but could spread the infection nonetheless. The more dangerous aspect of Dr. Francis' perspective is that we do not know whether there are differences in the viral strain that causes AIDS. There are known strain differences with other retroviruses. We do not know, however, if HTLV-III strain differences mean that further exposure to more or higher doses of different virus strains might further immunocompromise an individual, making an asymptomatic antibody positive person go on to develop full-blown AIDS. At present, the only safe response is to adopt safer sexual practices in society generally. Until we have effective immunomodulators and/or antiviral therapies, and a vaccine to prevent the access of the virus in noninfected persons, the best thing we can do is to educate people about the disease and appropriate preventive measures.

One other troubling factor relates to our knowledge about similar viruses. Some people suggest that an antibody, rather than a specific antigen test, is all that is required for public health purposes because retroviruses such as HTLV-III remain intracellular so that an exposed host is presumed to be infectious for life. This is relatively well-supported by our knowledge of the feline leukemia virus model. This retrovirus is known to stay with the cat until the cat dies, when the virus can be recovered. However, viral cultures are not invariably positive in all persons who have antibodies to HTLV-III, so we cannot invariably know who is infectious and who is not at this point in time on the basis of existing technologies.

The manner in which the tests for antibody to the virus are performed, or how viruses are grown in cell cultures, does not necessarily replicate the situation when two people are intimately kissing or having other kinds of contact. One has to be conservative, in light of the enormous, personal impact of a finding of a positive antibody test, in recommending alterations in patterns of intimate behavior, or stating unequivocally that a given behavior may or may not be safe. There are many things we still do not know about the virus and its transmission, *e.g.*, critical inoculum or the risks of "safer" sexual practices such as kissing. As better therapeutics become available for some of the other viruses such as Epstein-Barr virus and cytomegalovirus, it will be useful to know if patients with AIDS-related symptoms are actively infected with these other viruses. Therapeutic advances in the treatment of these other viral syndromes may improve the prognosis for persons with AIDS. Specific HTLV-III and other viral antibody tests may assist in following the clinical progression of specific viral infections in AIDS.

Appropriately developed learning programs for persons who want to take the ELISA test should be designed to inform the subject of the implications and limitations of the test. If this is done in a sensitive manner, behavioral theory would suggest that the experience could result in major behavior modification, *i.e.*, simply by undergoing a full educational program about the test, one could learn risk reduction. The data for this presumption are scant, and different centers have differing notions of what constitutes safe sex and how one should be counseled about the test. I have some difficulty with the concept of using testing as an educational tool in all cases because it implies a degree of paternalism and creates a potentially manipulative procedure. However, if properly utilized, administration of the test as a teaching device for purposes of behavior modification may be very useful. There are individuals who have told me that after having received test results (and I have heard this from people who have been negative and people who have been positive) that the testing process brought the epidemic much closer to home. It assisted them in addressing and resolving issues that later allowed them to change behavioral patterns which are, as we know, very difficult to change.

I have encountered other situations in which HTLV-III antibody screening has become a serious issue. Several women have talked to me about artificial insemination. These women had very close friends who were gay men and they wanted to know whether the test would be a useful adjunct in determining if it would be dangerous to receive sperm from these men. In counseling the women, I stressed that it was very important for them to have very candid relationships with those men. I explained that all individuals who are homosexually active do not have the same degree of risk, since they do not have the same sexual history. In terms of the test's predictive value in individuals who are at high risk for AIDS, a positive test has significant predictive value. In individuals who are at low risk for AIDS, the predictive value of a positive test is not as useful. Thus, I felt that I had to answer the women's questions with a somewhat relativistic answer. I suggested that if these men had positive tests, it would be necessary to have them not donate semen because of the attendant risk. If the tests were negative, I do not think the women could be completely reassured because of the potential risk that the men already were infected with the virus, but have not yet mounted an antibody response. Serial testing might be considered. The Red Cross guideline is that homosexually active males should not donate blood or semen because both are equally risky body fluids. These are the kinds of issues that are arising in a series of different, unpredictable situations. Thus, boycotting the test per se may not be feasible in everyone's life.

In another situation, a young man with generalized lymphadenopathy and profound malaise was unable to work. Social Security did not want to keep him on disability for more than six months in light of the presumed mononucleosis diagnosis, which should have resolved. More information on this medical condition was requested. The patient said this to me: "They implied that if I told [Social Security] that my physician was of the opinion that I might have ARC and could die from it, then they might be more willing to give me further disability." We discussed this approach at length and I was concerned about providing HTLV-III antibody results and other information to a federal agency. He felt that it was too difficult for him to get by without the financial assistance, and this difficulty outweighed his concerns about confidentiality. These are some of the difficulties that must be dealt with at the present time.

In Boston, we are performing epidemiologic studies at the Fenway Community Health Center in an effort to establish the risks of homosexually active men for developing AIDS. In the past we have had a great deal of enthusiasm and support for this type of research. Lately, there has been a "chill" over the work, primarily resulting from the manner in which the issues have been framed in recent months. A complicating factor relates to the directives from the federal government that projects funded by the federal government should inform individuals of the results of their tests. There are significant numbers of people who are willing to participate in studies to advance the state of scientific knowledge but are not interested in their test results. The gay community has become increasingly alienated by federal policies (such as routine military screening) which utilize the test as a diagnostic and prognostic tool and which could compromise their lifestyle and livelihood.

These policies raise serious ethical questions for the researcher. Is there a duty to warn others about high risk behavior in HTLV-III antibody positive persons? If a person has the antibody and remains active with new partners, what are the risks to other people and what is the investigator's role? We still do not fully know how to interpret the test, so the ethical responsibility of the clinician and researcher remains unclear. However, safe sex education is appropriate for seropositive and seronegative persons. Are we creating a biased sample of the high risk population if the only people who are willing to participate in research are those who are not concerned about learning the results? It is not clear what this bias will be. But this additional difficulty will have to be considered in interpreting new data.

While I am involved in projects where people are being tested for HTLV-III antibodies, I think it is important that the research community show sensitivity to the problems that individuals from the high risk groups have. The research community and the federal government must be more willing to fund education, outreach, and support for the people who are subject to societal stigma. The federal government does not appear to be interested in trying to take the lead in decreasing the general discrimination against high risk groups. There are many areas in which the federal government could say, "We realize we have a national crisis on our hands. One thing we need is to support and develop the good will of the communities at risk as best we can." This approach certainly has not been in evidence. It tends to increase the polarization of people with and at-risk for AIDS, which I think impacts negatively on research as well as on clinical care. We need to work together to address this problem together and all work towards the common good.

Critical Blood Banking Issues

Peter Page, M.D.
Director, American Red Cross Blood Services,
Northeast Region
Member, Mayor's and State Task Forces on
AIDS, Boston

The policies of the American Red Cross Blood Services towards patients and donors who test positive to HTLV-III antibodies are currently in a state of evolution. As we take actions relating to issues that arise from AIDS, we try to do so in a way that we can learn from our actions, so that mistakes will be minimized and that we can improve our policies as quickly as possible as we face issues that arise. I will discuss the policies and concerns about AIDS both for blood donors and for blood recipients. They relate to one another, but they are different.

In the blood banking area, remember that blood testing for *antibodies* to HTLV-III, the intent of which is to remove from the blood supply units potentially infectious for AIDS, is only one part of the many efforts already taken to make the blood supply safe from AIDS. In the same manner hepatitis B surface antigen testing (a specific and sensitive test for hepatitis B infectivity) is only one small part in minimizing post-transfusion hepatitis B. The most effective measure in maintaining the safety of the blood supply is the reliance upon volunteers, altruistic donors whose intent is to help, and not harm, others. Even with the anti-HTLV-III test, the most important measure to decrease transmission of AIDS, by blood transfusion, organ transplantation, or tissue implantation, remains the cooperation of volunteer members of the public. With rare exception, volunteer donors are honest and complete in providing medical history, and cooperate in deferring themselves, or being deferred by the Red Cross, from donating when appropriate. This test provides an additional increment of safety in that regard.

Concern has been expressed about false-positives and false-negatives in testing for anti-HTLV-III. It is important to reemphasize that the purpose of the test is to remove from the blood supply units that are potentially infectious. In order to most effectively remove the units that might be potentially infectious, the cutoff level for the difference between positive and negative test results has been purposefully put at a low point to maximize the usefulness of the test for its stated purpose and thereby include as many of the potentially infectious units as possible. By doing so, out of necessity one purposefully and artificially increases the false-positivity rate, an area of concern for donors but not for transfusion recipients. The intent of the test, in this setting, however, is to prevent transmission of AIDS by transfusion. A necessary, yet unfortunate, result is that by informing donors, or by providing information to donors that they are positive, they may, in fact, be falsely positive. On balance, this risk is determined to be less of a concern than not having this questionably infected donor seek further evaluation. That has been felt to be a lesser risk in this situation.

It has been previously stated and recommended by an interagency group and by a number of institutions that donors to be tested should be told prior to donating blood that they will be tested, and that if positive, they will be so informed and their names will be placed on a donor deferral register. The option of not being informed is not felt to be appropriate in the blood donor setting. Accordingly, if a person does not wish to learn his results, he should not donate. When we notify donors that they are positive, we need to minimize the harm to these donors since a significant percentage of them are likely to be falsely positive. We may be instilling long-lasting, serious, and unnecessary harm. When this test is performed, and as we inform donors of the results, it is our responsibility to provide to them all the information that we have that bears upon the test, its potential for false-positivity, and its potential for true-positivity. These volunteer donors, who are giving of themselves to help others, should have access to counseling and medical assistance. When we find donors to be positive, we should give them the opportunity, and encourage them, to enter into research programs so as to learn more about what being positive with this test means. If one is not in a risk group for AIDS, we need to learn whether there are other tests we can perform, other important epidemiologic factors or questions we can ask that could better determine the course of HTLV-III positivity. Perhaps we will learn of additional risk groups for AIDS, or perhaps learn other ways for determining which individuals are falsely positive. Donors testing positive should be regularly followed over at least a five-year period. There are a number of such studies being planned in regional blood centers in the United States. In Massachusetts, we have the support of the Massachusetts Department of Public Health in the initial funding of a study that addresses these areas. One benefit to this study is that by enrolling these donors in this research program, we can also readily give them access to counseling and other support services in the state. The development of the alternative testing site program has of necessity created a resource list of professionals who are informed and adept in these issues. We hope to use these experts for training staff, to provide information to test-positive donors, and to develop further our lists of interested and qualified professionals.

Another concern for regional blood centers and blood recipients is whether we will have enough blood donors to maintain the appropriate level of safe blood for the Commonwealth's use. Our foremost concern is that the blood supply be safe; in light of the very low chances of infecting a patient now, an overriding concern is that the blood supply remain adequate in amount. It is important that healthy persons not at risk for AIDS continue to donate, in spite of the fact that they will be tested. There have been estimates that as much as 5% of the population might discontinue donating blood because they do not want to be found to be positive or falsely positive. This is another major concern for us. We also need to reemphasize to the public that one cannot contract AIDS by donating blood. Blood needs to be available for transfusions before it is actually needed. One cannot donate blood for a friend or relative when the need becomes apparent; it needs to have been donated in advance since testing and processing must be completed prior to transfusion and take about a day. Sometimes, blood must be available in unexpectedly large amounts for a single patient. This demonstrates the necessity of having community blood donors giving blood regularly to ensure its availability for the unanticipated needs of any member of the community.

A major disadvantage of the AIDS epidemic and another area of concern is that there could be a decrease in blood donations as the public becomes aware that the donors will be tested and, if testing positive, will be told so, and placed on a donor deferral list. The people who have been blood donors have trusted the regional blood collecting agencies to maintain their confidentiality. That trust cannot be undermined. Donors accept some risks in being identified as false-positive; however, the impact of not having blood available when needed immediately to save a life is tremendous, so we need to continue our efforts to insure that that won't happen. Since donors have had trust in the agencies to which they have provided blood, to monitor and to look over the blood supply, then it is important that we continue to act in a way to preserve that trust. Regional blood collecting agencies have an excellent record of maintaining donor information in a confidential manner and utilizing it for the sole purpose of providing useful information to the donor and providing safe products for the recipients.

Blood donor information is not the same as a patient record or medical information. One can discuss the nature of the blood donor relationship; it can be stated as a participant volunteer relationship or as a contract. Regional blood services have not seen themselves historically as the health care providers of the donors. We manage the blood resource that the public voluntarily donates; in response to the donors' helping the community, we provide information concerning the testing of their blood donation which could be useful to them. They are referred on to other sources for medical care. The record to date for maintenance of confidentiality concerning hepatitis and other information which blood donors tell us and we find out by testing their blood, has been excellent. Protection against breaches of confidentiality is taken very seriously by blood banking facilities. There is legislation being proposed on the federal level that would protect this information from subpoena. It is not so protected in all states at this time, however.

With respect to the risks to transfusion recipients, they need to be informed of the risks of transfusion. This is nothing new, as there are other serious risks of transfusion besides AIDS. For example, 5% of transfusion recipients develop evidence of non-A, non-B hepatitis infection. Usually, it is a mild disease, being subclinical and not noticed. Many years later, however, it may progress to cirrhosis. It has been estimated that every year in the United States 600 to 700 people die from other types of transfusion-associated hepatitis. We already have an excellent test for hepatitis B; there is another kind of hepatitis, non-A, non-B, for which there is no specific test. Other complications of blood transfusions can be due to the clerical error of giving a patient a "mismatched" unit or the "wrong" unit of blood.

At this time, there are approximately 130 patients with AIDS associated with blood transfusion. Without minimizing that number or its importance, consider it in light of other transfusion risks that the public and physicians have accepted. The media has provided us with an opportunity to remind patients and physicians of the risks of transfusions, and that people should not be unnecessarily transfused. However, the public needs to have reassurance that the blood supply is quite safe and that if they need transfusion, they should have transfusion. A phobia about AIDS should not interfere with the necessary transfusion of a patient; his life could be saved by it. A death brought on by refusing a blood transfusion clearly would be a worse problem than the very small risk of transfusion-associated AIDS, which is in the range of one in hundreds of thousands. Also, due to the long incubation period of this disease, the risk of being transfused today is much less than the risk several years ago before we were aware of this problem and before we solicited the cooperation of persons at risk from not donating blood.

There are other issues of transfusion recipients who have already been transfused. In our investigation of these hundred or so patients who developed AIDS from transfusions, we have questioned the donors. In going back to each group of donors whose blood went to a patient who seemed to get AIDS for no reason other than transfusion, in virtually every case, a high risk donor for AIDS has been identified. In the cases we have been investigating, all these donations occurred before 1983. Thus, those transfusions occurred before we knew there was a problem, and before persons at risk were encouraged not to donate.

When we learn that a patient has transfusion-associated AIDS, and one of the recipient's donors is at risk for AIDS, most of these donors, but not all, have remained healthy. Current practice in blood banking is to split a unit of whole blood into three parts immediately after the donation: red cells, platelets, and plasma. Each implicated donation could therefore also have resulted in two other products transfused to two other patients. Should those other two recipients of that unit be so notified? It has been the feeling of the major blood banking organizations that the blood collecting service should notify the blood transfusion service about that event. Typically, the clinician of those additional two recipients would be informed of the situation so that they might be alerted to the possibility of a contaminated transfusion. The question was raised as to whether it will be helpful to the individual to learn this information; because one was transfused with such a unit does not mean that the agent was transmitted, or that the recipient will get sick. This is one of the more difficult issues that we are dealing with. We inform most patients of these risks in order to minimize the risk of that person being lost to our surveillance and to assure good patient care through their clinician. We are interested in learning the outcome of such patients. Their physicians may want to perform further evaluations or give advice to these patients.

Prospective studies and research about such recipients are ongoing and are very helpful to us to assess the risks. Now that we have implemented anti-HTLV-III testing, if a donor is found to be anti-HTLV-III positive, we will discard the unit of blood. Typically, donors are allowed to donate every eight weeks. If the donor who is positive today donated eight weeks ago, then three patients from the earlier donation may have been transfused with that blood. Should those recipients be notified? Do we know that that person was positive eight weeks ago? This issue is made even more complicated by the lack of studies which correlate blood infectivity and transmissibility with anti-HTLV-III positivity. If we were to notify the recipients of this donation eight weeks ago, what about the recipient 16 weeks ago? The incubation period of AIDS is shown to be up to 62 months by the transfusion-associated data. Should we go back and notify all the recipients of all the donations for the last five years? The logistics and the paperwork are already a mammoth task. It is possible to do, but we currently lack the resources. By not knowing whether the person was anti-HTLV-III positive long ago, and not knowing whether they were infected at all, one can question the relative value of following that approach. There are those who would argue that a person who has been transfused may be at risk for AIDS, may be at a risk for hepatitis, and the knowledge by his clinician that he was transfused at all is enough to be more suspicious of any other conditions arising that may be related to AIDS. There is an argument not to notify such persons of the risk for developing AIDS. The anticipated risk to the recipient appears to be small although it is not yet well-quantified. One could offer anti-HTLV-III testing to past transfusion recipients who are interested in learning their status.

I think this points out, as was mentioned earlier, the importance of public education. It is important for us to minimize confusion and to make sure that physicians are aware of what is known and what is not known. I hope that we can act responsibly, to learn as much as we can as quickly as we can so that we can be more appropriate in our responses. We must keep an open mind to modify and improve these responses as we learn more.

Question

If the HTLV-III antibody screening test is less predictive in low risk populations, if the test cannot distinguish between gay blood, straight blood, IV drug user blood, and if a higher level of false-positives in low risk people is assumed, then it sounds "homophobic" to me that we tell high risk people, "You have tested positive so you have to be careful" and yet to low risk people, "We do not really think you are at risk, don't worry about it too much." Is this based on the assumption that the test is less predictive in low risk people or is it another expression of a strong social bias?

Answer

What is closer to the reality of the HTLV-III test is that there are a certain number of persons who do not have the disease, yet their test results will actually be in the positive test area. Since the ELISA test gives a number rather than a yes or no answer, depending on where the line is drawn to differentiate positive from negative results, will determine the number of false-positives or false-negatives that result from the test. Ideally, a test that gives 100% separation between those who are test positive (and have the disease), and those who are test negative (and do not), is preferred. Such a perfect test is only rarely developed. If you draw the line for test positive or test negative all the way to one side, no false-negatives will result and all the positive persons that you want will be identified but along with a number of false-positives. A theoretical distribution of the results of two tested populations would reveal one population not having the disease, another population having the disease (or the infection), and an area of uncertainty in between which becomes more gray, where some people will test positive without the disease and vice versa. The understanding of the companies who developed the test was to draw their line somewhere in between, to minimize the number of false-positives, but more important for the safety of the blood supply to minimize the number of false-negatives, yet having a useful test that is somewhat predictive of infectivity. Remember that the issue here is infection with the virus, not the disease.

It is apparent that if you test a population which in fact is infected, then the number of false-positives will greatly decrease. If you test a population that does not have infection, the number of false-positives increases as the sample size increases. Theoretically, if a population has no infection, they could have a 50% false-positive rate. There is probably a 50% false-positive rate in the population that has very little infection; if a population carries the infection, in fact, the false-positive rate is considerably less. I don't think this has anything to do with discrimination; I think it has to do with the biology of the virus and the nature of the test.

Question

I read a Defense Department Military Blood Program office memorandum addressed to the Surgeon Generals in the military which required all military and civilian blood agencies conducting blood drives on base to report any positive test results to appropriate military health agencies so that they may take preventive medical measures. While this is less of an issue now that the military will test for HTLV-III antibodies, will the American Red Cross participate in the military's directive?

Answer

In the Northeast Region (Maine and Massachusetts) we rely to a significant degree upon the military for voluntary blood donation, to the extent of about 20,000 pints of blood each year. We have not provided the results of any HTLV-III testing to the military. We provide some blood grouping information, such as ABO and Rh groups, to the military for recruitment purposes, but that is all. I have reemphasized to the local bases that it is our policy not to provide test result information except to the person being tested. This raises some delicate issues that hopefully can be resolved without undue loss of blood donors or confidentiality of the individuals.

An alternative, if it becomes necessary, is to inform prospective donors on military bases in advance of donating that, if positive, the information would be released to a physician. Currently, donor's hepatitis results are reported to a physician only with the donor's signed permission to do so in advance.

With respect to the issue of the reportability of test positivity, in Massachusetts and Maine, AIDS is a reportable condition; however, a positive test result is not reported. We have worked closely with these state departments of public health. Those states' departments agree that a positive test result alone does not constitute a disease or make a diagnosis, and does not need to be reported. We are not yet aware of the significance of a positive test result, and apart from education, at this point we are not really certain what proper public health measures should be taken in any event.

Accordingly, information concerning any donors found to be positive stays within the Red Cross system and does not get reported to the state. In Massachusetts, that is also the case for hepatitis B surface antigen tests.

Question

If blood banks are screening each unit with what appears to be a fairly sensitive test, and if the people are not taking part in a long-term surveillance study, what exactly is the point of keeping a "deferral" list?

Answer

We provide pamphlets of information to all prospective donors before they are tested. Donors are told that if they test positive, they will be so informed and that their names will be put on a donor deferral registry list. They certify that they have read and understand the information pamphlet, which serves as the informed consent.

The purpose of keeping the deferral list is to exclude from transfusion, units subsequently donated from people who are on the list. Any subsequent units so identified are also destroyed. If such a person donates blood again, he or she is checked against the deferral list and tested again.

A concern has been raised that a person may convert from positive to negative over time. We do not have any scientific support evidence in donors to this argument. Also, perhaps the lots of test reagent vary and the viral titer in the individual can vary. Even in the best of all worlds, errors will be made. In order to protect blood recipients, however, we will discard a unit from a person who was tested earlier and found to be positive, as we have done with hepatitis for many years.

As an aside, deferral lists are kept within an individual collecting agency, as required by federal law. For example, if Hospital A collects blood from a donor, Hospital A keeps its list to itself. The Red Cross system is considered to be a single collecting facility and shares this list within its own system. We have recently modified this list so that if a donor donates in one Red Cross center and is found to be positive and put on the list, and subsequently donates in another center, the other center will know only in checking the list that the blood should not be transfused. They will not know why. AIDS, hepatitis, HTLV-III positivity, malaria, or other conditions could cause the donor's name to be placed on the donor list. The reason is kept locally and does not go to other local centers.

Question

I am not certain that most people are aware that the Centers for Disease Control (CDC) has finally dropped Haitians from the list of people at high risk for AIDS. Neither the CDC nor the media has actively informed the public about the decision, which was a useful exercise in epidemiologic research. Haitian physicians in North America convinced the CDC, after much discussion, to perform epidemiologic studies on the Haitians in North America. Two places were considered, New York and Miami. The first study included 100 healthy Haitians, some departing Haiti before and some after 1977. HTLV-III tests were performed; none of the persons was found to have a positive test.

Another study involved 58 Haitian patients and 300 Haitians matched for lifestyle and associated in other relevant parameters. Of the 300 people, six of them were found to have positive HTLV-III titers. The CDC finally agreed that Haitian nationals do not present a risk higher than non-Haitians.

As of April, 1985, the National Red Cross used a questionnaire for prospective blood donors and listed that anyone who has been in Haiti or Zaire should not be considered a viable candidate to donate blood. What are the scientific grounds for this distinction? Shouldn't the Red Cross revise their questionnaire to exclude all donors who have lived in New York and California?

Answer

I wish I had a complete explanation for this. This is an area of great concern to me and, really, to the Red Cross. We have a deep concern for the health of prospective blood donors. Our overriding concern, however, is to protect the recipients of the donated blood. Red Cross tends to be zealously cautious and protective of the quality of the blood supply. It takes time to alter national policy for an entity with this perspective. I should point out that persons visiting these and many other areas in the last three years are likely to be deferred in any event for reasons concerning potential malaria exposure.

Question

I am concerned about the issue of discrimination resulting from the use of HTLV-III results. I recently listened to a so-called "Christian" physician on national radio who gave a special report on AIDS. He called for a national quarantine of all members in the risk groups, all the current AIDS patients, and everyone who tests positive to HTLV-III. While this is an extremist's perspective, it is important to note that these crazy people are out there and often are heard faster in Washington than you or me. The people with false-positive and true-positive results may never become ill. How should these issues of discrimination and lack of scientific certainty be addressed?

Answer

(Alvin Novick, M.D.): I think that AIDS is exacerbating many of the underlying tensions in the health care delivery system. As we learn more about the disease, we will be able to make more informed decisions. The state of the scientific art does not allow us to interpret, in a definitive manner, the results of the test. It is the best that we have, though, and it is highly improper to say, "Let's ignore the test and the implications of the test." Another serious problem is balancing the risk of AIDS to people receiving blood with the risk of social disability to blood donors. Perhaps 50 to 100 people will develop AIDS from transfusions this year. The test may cause 20,000 to 40,000 donors to address the question of the implications of a positive test. Will they fear having children or having sex with their spouse? Will their spouse's fear of having sex with them lead to divorce and to unmarriageability? Such people may belong to low risk groups with very little social support. Gay men, while they have little support from the general public, have very strong support from their own communities. Other donors at low risk, while they have excellent support from the general public, will not have support from family, friends, or the general public. We clearly need public advocates for the blood donor, especially because those blood donors are essential for health care in this country.

As we implement this test, we need to provide access for counseling and other support systems for donors and others with positive test results.

Comment

(Mathilde Krim, M.D.): The test is not foolproof. A certain proportion of the results are false-positives; other results are false-negatives. In terms of medical problems and the test having its major use in the screening of blood, it is the false-negative results which are most worrisome. Even if applied under the best laboratory conditions, we will miss the virus being present in some units of blood. The blood will remain, to a certain extent, contaminated.

The false-negative results are mostly due to the fact that following infection, antibodies to the virus do not develop immediately. They appear between one month and six months after infection. If a person is tested for antibody before the antibody appears, the result will be a "false" negative, even though the person is actively infected. The person's blood would be contagious and, if donated, would be routed into the blood supply for transfusion. Nothing at this time, except the social screening procedures, is available to stop this unit of blood from entering the system.

Some individuals who are tested do not want to be told of the test result, the so-called "right not to know." I concluded that a person may have a right not to be administered the test; however, once the test is administered that person now has an obligation to society, to his friends, family, and lovers, to modify his or her behavior where a positive test dictates. The people performing the tests and informing the donor or other tested person must provide appropriate counseling. For quite a while, the AIDS Medical Foundation, for example, did not advise people at risk to take the test. We felt that the risk due to possible breaks in confidentiality were too significant when balanced against the advantages of knowing the test results. It has become apparent that concern about protection of confidentiality has increased; certain measures have been taken in New York City, for example. The New York City Health Department, which now provides the test at an alternative site, has made provision to protect confidentiality by using certain statutes that allow complete protection of confidentiality of people involved in research. Under this umbrella of protection, the Health Department provides the test and will not disclose the name of the participants. Perhaps now, the AIDS Medical Foundation in New York should modify our position, encouraging testing.

The Gift of Blood: Social Policy in Evolution

Johanna Pindyck, M.D.
Vice President, New York Blood Center
Director, Greater New York Blood Program

In 1982, the first cases of AIDS in hemophilia patients and transfusion recipients were identified. This led to the recognition that AIDS is a blood-transmissible disease. This, in turn, led to the need to protect the safety of the blood supply for recipients, and required responses which directly affect and potentially or actually infringe upon the rights of blood donors. Early in 1985, the screening of all donated blood for donor exposure to the HTLV-III virus, the causative agent of AIDS, was introduced by blood collection agencies throughout the United States and abroad. Socially acceptable measures had to be devised rapidly to protect the rights of recipients to a safe blood supply without unduly violating the rights of donors.

What rights of privacy and confidentiality do blood donors have, and what responsibilities fall on the shoulders of blood collection agencies in order to protect these rights? I propose that there are six major rights of blood donors: the donors have a right to give blood, a right to privacy, a right to make an informed decision to give that blood, a right to take risks, a right to be protected from harm, and a right to receive information of importance to personal or public health. Many of these rights are influenced by public health policy, and by the recipient's primary right to a safe blood supply. I have attempted to examine these rights in this context.

The individual has a right to give blood. Individuals who wish to give blood, do so either as volunteer unpaid donors, as are almost all of the whole blood donors in the United States, or for money, as are almost all of the plasma donors in the United States. Both groups have had restrictions imposed on their right to give blood for a long time, depending on their health and medical history. The purpose of these restrictions is to protect the public's, the donor's, and the recipient's safety. Similar restrictions exist in many other areas of our society. For example, I have the right to drive, but I must wear my glasses. My uncorrected vision is sufficiently impaired to endanger my safety and that of others if I were to drive without them. With the recognition of AIDS as a blood-transmissible disease, epidemiologic evidence requires the exclusion of members of the AIDS risk groups as blood donors in our society. Many of these individuals have previously been permitted to give blood, and concern was expressed in some quarters that this restriction was tantamount to discrimination. It is to the credit of the leadership of organizations that represent AIDS risk group members that they have recognized the medical necessity of this step and actively support the introduction of socially acceptable ways to accomplish this goal.

These "socially acceptable" measures had to respect another right of the donor—the donor's right to privacy. How has this been accomplished? Since 1983, in the United States, all prospective blood and plasma donors have been given information about groups at risk for contracting AIDS and have been asked not to give blood if they were members of these groups. This is a private decision of the donor. Some blood collection agencies have also added a procedure that permits persons in risk groups who might feel that this request not to donate compromises their rights of privacy to give blood. These donors may confidentially advise the collection agency that their donation should be used for laboratory studies only, and not for patient transfusion. A form is completed by all donors in order to afford this opportunity to all donors in a confidential manner. The donor indicates his or her decision, requesting that the donation be used only for study or may be used for transfusion. The form is sealed by the donor privately. Privacy issues are currently of paramount importance for blood collection agencies, as they relate to the need to maintain confidentiality of results of anti-HTLV-III screening of the donated blood.

What about the right to make an informed decision to donate? Within the health care field, blood collection agencies have been somewhat late in recognizing the importance of this right. The issues surrounding the introduction of anti-HTLV-III screening have had a salutary effect and have heightened our awareness of the need to respect this right. I would remind you, however, that it was only 20 years ago that the medical profession and the general public had little concern for informed consent. Instead, release forms were used, the primary purpose of which was to protect hospitals and physicians from liability. The situation has now changed in health care, and is currently undergoing change in blood collection procedures. Socially conscious individuals, bioethicists, legislators, regulators, attorneys, health care practitioners, and the courts have been powerful agents for social reform in the informed consent area in health care; the same is true now with respect to blood donation.

In exploring this issue at a recent meeting of the American Blood Commission, Nancy Dubler, an attorney affiliated with Montefiore Hospital in New York City and the Hastings Center in Hastings-on-Hudson in New York, viewed the relationship between the donor and the blood collection agency as a contract. The donor donates blood to the agency. In exchange, the blood collection agency sets forth and informs the donor of the terms of the contract, including the agency's duties relating to confidentiality. Acceptance by the donor of the terms is indicated by a signed consent for the donation. Although breach of contract actions in the health care setting have not been upheld, in general, by the courts, this particular approach may cause courts to reconsider the contract notion in the blood bank setting.

Many people have been concerned about the personal and societal risks of anti-HTLV-III testing. What about the donor's right to take risks? I would suggest that society is permissive with respect to the right of individuals to take risks. Judging by the conclusions of philosophers, ethicists, and the courts, and as stated by the Christian ethicist, Paul Ramsey, when discussing medical research, "No consent, rather than no risk, or no discernible risk, is the decisive point at law and in morality."[1] I believe the same holds true for blood donation and many other activities in which we choose to engage, as long as an informed choice is made.

The last two rights I would like to discuss are the donor's right to be protected from harm and to receive information of importance to his or her personal and public health. I have combined them together deliberately: donors have the right to be protected from harm during and after a blood donation. Medical screening, caution during the collection itself, and observation during the rest period are three ways in which blood collection agencies seek to protect this right of the donor. In addition, strict protection of information about the donor, including the protection of his or her laboratory test result, except as required under public health law and hopefully so stated to the donor, is another example.

Presently, blood collection agencies are struggling with another issue related both to the donor's right to protection from harm and to the right to receive information of importance to health. This issue relates to the handling of anti-HTLV-III screening reactive test results. As I noted, blood collection agencies are performing anti-HTLV-III screening of donated blood. In fact, many, including the Greater New York Blood Program, are already testing all donated blood. In New York, that amounts to testing of 2,200 volunteer donor units each day. These samples are tested even though we know that a large percentage, as many as 50% to 90% of the reactive samples on screening, will be falsely positive. We withdraw these reactive units from the blood supply to safeguard blood recipients. Should we tell the donors of reactive results, knowing that 50% to 90% are false-positives? Should we test further and try to define the positive reactions and notify only those donors? If one of the rights of donors is protection from harm, it is critical that we determine whether one would do harm to a person by informing him or her of a test reaction which is not really an indicator of AIDS virus exposure in that person. AIDS is a lethal disease which strikes terror in the mind of the public. Can we expect donors to cope with information about false-positive reactions when physicians are themselves unclear on this issue? Some public health officials advocate the release of information on screening reactive donors. Others do not. Many of us in the blood bank community believe that considerable harm would come to individuals advised of falsely positive screen reactive results. Except within approved research guidelines, public health officials, biomedical scientists, blood bankers, ethicists, sociologists, and others are currently struggling to resolve this very pressing issue. As you see, I hope, the gift of blood is truly a social policy in evolution.

Question

You mentioned that the ELISA test led to 50% to 90% biologic false-positives. It is my understanding that the ELISA test being licensed by the FDA leads to a 0.1% biologic false-positive. Could you explain this discrepancy?

Answer

My comment about the false-positives relates specifically to the performance of the test in the donor population. The data on the specificity and sensitivity of the test, however, are derived from data on patients with AIDS or lymphadenopathy syndrome. When the ELISA test is used as a screening test in a non-ill population, one has a totally different situation. If you read the manufacturer's instructions from the licensed kit, both Ambit and NML, they speak directly to the issue of 50% to 90% false-positives when the test is used as a screening test in the donor population. People who meet the CDC definition for AIDS will test positive almost 100% of the time. Healthy blood donors with no risk factors for exposure to HTLV-III are approximately 99.3% test negative. Of the 0.7% who have tested positive, where the Western blot or other more sensitive tests are used, 0.3% or so will be true-positives, and 0.4% will be false-positives. If one were to donate, the specificity of the test is 99.3%; however, of those people who test positive by the kit, half (or more) will be false-positive results. The blood banking community is seriously concerned about the questions that false-positives raise. Approximately eight million people donate blood each year in the United States. If roughly 1% of the people screened with the ELISA test are reactive, and 50% of these people are falsely positive, then we have the potential of 40,000 individuals who could be notified that they have tested "positive" when, in effect, the result is erroneous. The use of confirmatory testing in this population is essential, but it is inordinately expensive, time consuming, and very slow.

Research Risks and Federally-Funded Studies

F. William Dommel, Jr.
Assistant Director, Office for Protection from
Research Risks, National Institutes of Health

The Office for Protection from Research Risks, in the Office of the Director of the National Institutes of Health (NIH), is responsible for the development, implementation, and provision of compliance oversight of regulations designed for the protection of human research subjects in research that is funded by the Department of Health and Human Services and carried out primarily in the Centers for Disease Control (CDC) and the NIH. The regulations that were first published in 1974, and significantly revised in 1981, are the product of years of study and public debate. The adequate protection of human subjects in research demands adherence to the following principles in the conduct of all research. First, the substantive respect for all persons, that individuals be regarded as autonomous agents, that those with diminished autonomy be provided additional protections, and that a subject in a research study must be totally informed of the research risks in order to participate in research. Second, the principle of beneficence is that one must ensure that the benefits of research are maximized, and that the risks of harm are to be minimized. Third, justice demands the equitable distribution of benefits and the equitable selection of subjects.

When the Public Health Service and the Office for the Protection from Research Risks began to review the proposed testing of blood for HTLV-III antibodies, these principles of respect for persons, beneficence, and justice remained of paramount importance in the design of any study. The human subject protection regulations, set forth at 45 CFR Part 46, apply these three principles by requiring that institutions applying for support for research involving human subjects file an assurance of compliance with the regulations. The National Research Act of 1974 required that the Secretary of the department of Health and Human Services issue regulations requiring that any institution conducting research involving human subjects and funded by the department establish Investigational Review Boards (IRB), the approval of which would be a prerequisite to the conduct of any research funded by the department. Nearly all major research institutions in the United States follow these rules for all research, not just that conducted through the support of the Department of Health and Human Services, but without regard to source of funding. The regulations require that the IRBs be established in the following manner: (1) there must be at least five persons of varying backgrounds on the board qualified to evaluate the research; (2) the IRB members must be sensitive to community attitudes; (3) one member must be a nonscientist; (4) one member must not be affiliated with the institution; (5) one member must be a man; (6) one member must be a woman; and, (7) if an IRB regularly reviews research involving vulnerable populations, the IRB shall include one or more persons concerned with the welfare of those subjects. These regulations should be kept in mind in the AIDS research (and nonresearch) area, because they are particularly applicable. An IRB regularly reviewing research involving AIDS patients should include members who are advocates for those who suffer from hemophilia.

Within these duties described above are several functions that are particularly important to AIDS studies. In an evaluation of a human research study, an IRB is required to address confidentiality twice. Where appropriate, the IRB must make the determination that there are adequate provisions to protect the privacy of subjects, and to maintain the confidentiality of the data. In the evaluation of the informed consent process, including the document of informed consent to be signed by a research subject, informed consent must include a statement to the research subject describing the extent, if any, to which confidentiality of records identifying the subject will be maintained. Next, the subject must be fully informed of the degree to which confidentiality will be maintained. Confidentiality is a crucial issue, drawing and deserving the closest scrutiny possible by an IRB.

There are two pertinent exemptions to the IRB regulations. The first exemption relates to all survey interviews and observational research projects. Survey interviews and observational research projects are not exempt, however, if all of the following three conditions are met: (1) if the identity of the individual will be recorded, or identifiers that could be linked to the individual will be recorded; (2) if the subject's responses becoming known outside the research project could reasonably place the subject at risk of criminal or civil liability, or be damaging to the subject's financial standing or employability; and (3) if the research deals with sensitive aspects of human behavior, such as illegal conduct, drug use, sexual behavior, or use of alcohol.

When these regulations were issued, the exemptions were declared by the secretary as being categories of research which, in the opinion of the secretary, represented little or no risk to research subjects. If these three conditions are met, however, and in nearly all AIDS research involving "surveys, interviews, or observations of public behavior," these three conditions are met, then AIDS research would not be exempt from the regulations, even though most other survey and interview research is exempt.

This is rather distressing news. Careful consideration of the human subject protections regulations, and careful application of these rules did occur throughout the development of the HTLV-III antibody screening kits. Our office issued advisory information to IRBs in December, 1984 about this issue which attempted to guide IRBs through the difficult thought processes.

The confidentiality considerations applicable to research on AIDS patients are also critical in nonresearch settings, where they should provide a useful framework and guideline for evaluating problems in the AIDS area.

References

1. Ramsey, P. 1970. *The Patient As Person*. New Haven: Yale University Press.

PART VII
Cultural and Historical Perspectives

Historical Analogies to the AIDS Epidemic

Allan M. Brandt, Ph.D.
Assistant Professor of the History of Medicine and Science
Harvard Medical School

In looking at the current situation of AIDS, it is impossible not to be struck by many analogies with the history of venereal disease in the 20th century. These analogies relate to science, public health, and especially to social and cultural values.

The manner in which a society responds to a disease, and especially to those in need, reveals very deep and fundamental cultural and social values. A disease is shaped not only by its biological qualities, but by cultural variables as well. A disease can become a symbol for ordering and explaining various aspects of human experience. Medicine and science are not only affected by social, economic, and political variables; medicine and science are, in fact, embedded in them. This has been particularly true in the 20th century relating to sexually transmitted diseases. These diseases have been put to various social and political uses. They have served various functions in our society, many of which we should be gravely concerned about. At the very least, we should remember how they have been used.

Generally, these diseases have been used as a means of indicating a corrupt sexuality, or to identify those who were seen as willfully violating a particular moral code. They have been seen as a punishment, be it just or unjust, for those who were sexually irresponsible. Sexually transmitted diseases are typically viewed as diseases of behavior. This characterization distinguishes them in certain ways from other diseases, although there are, of course, other diseases that are also emphasized as being behavioral in nature.

Because they are seen, as Susan Sontag has indicated, as a metaphor for evil and sin, this has led to powerful stigma towards those who contract these diseases.[1] It is also important to consider, when we think about metaphors or symbols relating to various diseases, that these are not only symbols or some kind of linguistic construction. These symbols have a powerful impact on public health interventions, medical interventions, and the manner in which doctors confront patients.

At the turn of the 20th century, there was a very similar hysteria regarding syphilis and gonorrhea not unlike what we are experiencing today with AIDS. There were a number of reasons why the so-called "progressives" of that era thought venereal disease was an indication of social disorder. They were gravely concerned about the growth of the cities, the revolution in science and technology, and the influx of immigrants from foreign lands. At this time, a redefinition of the social meaning of venereal disease took place. It went from being what physicians and lay people called the "carnal scourge," a punishment for moral misbehavior, to being referred to as a "family poison." These changes were also fundamentally related to changes in the biomedical sciences. Important discoveries by German and French researchers about the existence and transmissibility of the infectious organisms affected social behavior considerably.

People began to realize that men who visited prostitutes, for example, could come home and infect their wives and their children. Many individuals became blinded during childbirth by the infectious organism that causes gonorrhea. As late as 1915, although there were methods for preventing these types of infection, as many as 25% of all the blind in the United States had become blind by ophthalmia neonatorum, or gonorrheal blindness. Also, physicians became very concerned about sterility in women because it was felt that they could not reproduce in sufficient numbers if they became sterile due to these venereal diseases. In fact, there was a famous Broadway play in 1913 called *Damaged Goods,* that told the story of a man about to be married who visited a prostitute and spread disease in this manner.

At that time, physicians also began to discuss what they called "syphilis of the innocent" or casually transmitted venereal disease. They suggested that individuals could contract veneral diseases by everyday activities and without sexual contact. These instances of venereal disease were widely reported in the medical literature. One physician who wrote the definitive textbook on venereal diseases wrote, "The methods by which non-venereal syphilis may be acquired are innumerable and relate to every conceivable circumstance surrounding life."[2]

Physicians began to catalogue the various ways that syphilis might be communicated, including such things as pens, pencils, toothbrushes, or tatoos. To give one indication of how seriously this was taken, during the First World War, the Navy removed all the door knobs off its battleships. It was suggested that this was a way many sailors might be getting their infections. When physicians became infected, it was usually suggested that this happened during surgical procedures on patients with venereal diseases.

The following excerpt of a short story by a woman who became infected in one of these ways indicates the social concern about venereal diseases early in the 20th century.

At first it was unbelievable. I knew of the disease only through newspaper advertisements [for patent medicines for venereal disease]. I'd understood that it was the result of sin, and originated and was contracted only in the underworld of the city. I felt sure that my friend was mistaken in diagnosis when he exclaimed, "another tragedy of the public drinking cup." I eagerly met his remark with assurance that I did not use public drinking cups, that I'd used my own drinking cup for summers. He led me to review my summer. After recalling a number of times when my thirst had forced me to go to the public fountain, I came at last to realize that what he had told me was true.[3]

This story was written at a time when public fountains had a chain with a metal drinking cup attached. One of the few public health interventions that was undertaken at that time was by public health workers who went around clipping off these metal drinking cups in places like the Boston Common because it was feared that this was a mechanism for spreading venereal diseases.

It is interesting to consider what might be the impact of this notion that venereal disease could be spread through nonsexual contacts. One might surmise that this could lead to an opening up of treatment programs, that this might lead to the notion that venereal diseases are like any other diseases—people can get them in many ways without moral indiscretion, and therefore, a public health response might be considered. The woman who wrote this story had an interesting reaction that was not uncharacteristic. She wrote, "If each state would pass and enforce stringent laws causing persons so diseased to be isolated just as lepers are, there would be more hope in repressing the evil."[3] This type of response reflects a concern about the heterogeneity of American society. At a time when a pluralistic culture was becoming a significant aspect of American life, there was grave concern about notions of contamination, filth, and hygiene, all reflected in this fear that venereal disease could be transmitted in a variety of ways. It was soon discovered, however, that syphilis and gonorrhea could not be transmitted in this manner.

This perspective raises a number of concerns about the way venereal disease is viewed, and the way contacts among different peoples are viewed. There was a well-known gynecologist at Johns Hopkins University, Dr. Howard Kelly, who was one of the leading figures in American medicine in the early 20th century. He wrote:

> The personal services of the poor must daily invade our doors and penetrate every nook in our houses. If we care for them in no wise beyond their mere service to us, woe betide us. Think of these countless currents flowing daily in our cities from the houses of the poorest into those of the richest and forming a sort of civic circulatory system expressive of the life of the body politic. A circulation which continually tends to equalize the distribution of morality and disease.

I think that the situation with AIDS in the last few years has again raised this notion of fear of contamination, fear of unhygienic sexuality that reflects, in part, an alien notion of impurity or of taboo acts. It is very interesting to see this response, because even in responsible assessments of the AIDS crisis, there have been these kinds of suggestions. In 1983, in the *New York Times Magazine,* this question was raised in an analogous fashion:

The groups most recently found to be at risk for AIDS present a particularly poignant problem. Innocent bystanders caught in the path of a new disease. They can make no behavioral decisions to minimize their risk. Hemophiliacs cannot stop taking blood clotting medication, surgery patients cannot stop getting transfusions, women cannot control the drug habits of their mates, babies cannot choose their mothers.

What I am suggesting is that values—cultural and social values—that get involved in assessments of problems of disease, can be very subtle and very difficult to discern. This for the most part was a responsible, clear account of the recent AIDS research. But it suggests that those victims who are not homosexual present a particularly poignant problem; the implication is that deaths from this disease among homosexuals are somewhat less poignant, less significant. Those who can make no behavioral decisions to minimize their risk are somehow more deserving of sympathy than those who can make behavioral decisions. Implicit in such formulations is a simplistic and naive view of human behavior.

There is a notion that this disease is, in fact, a behavioral problem that can be solved tl.rough a simple change of behavior. This has been the assumption concerning venereal disease throughout the 20th century. The public health and social perspective is why devote money to public health campaigns, or why spend money on clinical research relating to venereal diseases when this is a simple problem. It can be solved by changes in behavior. I would argue that this way of viewing disease—this social construction—has had a powerful effect on inhibiting a series of public health interventions that might have had a beneficial impact on sexually transmitted diseases in the 20th century. It raises equally important questions for us to consider when we think about the problem of AIDS. There has been a tremendous ambivalence within the medical world concerning the treatment of sexually transmitted diseases in the 20th century. As I researched the history of venereal disease, I was amazed to find that some physicians who had dedicated their lives to conquering these diseases, when finally presented with penicillin, an effective treatment for gonorrhea and especially for syphilis, were suddenly very concerned that the treatment that they had hoped for all of their lives would have a very deleterious impact on American sexual ethics. This is clearly documented in the medical literature.[6] It was as though they suggested that treatment for these diseases might create a problem worse than the disease itself. In this, the notion of the punitive quality of some of the venereal disease treatments that have been offered in the past becomes apparent.

The other question this raises relates to civil liberties, or the balance of the conflicting values of social good and individual responsibility. Who is responsible? What is the role of the individual? What are the rights of the individual and the rights of the community? There have been very powerful concerns about these issues relating to venereal disease which again go back to the turn of the 20th century. During the First World War, there was a massive attempt to arrest prostitutes because it was feared that they were spreading venereal disease to the troops. As many as 40,000 to 60,000 prostitutes were interned in camps, not unlike the camps that were constructed for Japanese-Americans during the Second World War. This little-known story reveals the concerns about communicability, contamination, and infectiousness.

The other issue it raises relates to the history of screening—another issue which has tremendous contemporary importance. Various tests were developed by scientists for screening venereal disease, especially the Wassermann test for syphilis. By 1935, many state legislatures began to pass laws that required people to take these tests before they could legally marry. It was later discovered—many years later—that the Wassermann test had a false-positive rate as high as 25%. A very large number of individuals were not permitted to marry and most probably suffered long and toxic treatments. Because this was before the promulgation of antibiotics in the 1940s, those who could not marry took arsenic treatments because they believed they had a serious disease. This raises questions about the relationship of science and social policy. What do we know and how do we begin to develop policies from the scientific answers that we have, insufficient as they often are?

This suggests my last question which relates to the issue of scientific uncertainty. For all the attention that AIDS has received in the last few years and for all the information that we now have, it seems that for every scientific fact that we may feel we understand about this problem, there is a host of problems that we don't understand. How do you make proper public policy or address a question when much is not understood? In times of scientific uncertainty, there is a great tendency to fill the scientific vacuum with the social and cultural values which prevail. There may be significant attempts to segment society around an issue of social value rather than to see this as a problem of American society which needs to be addressed in a central way. Until we more fully recognize the ways in which social and cultural values and attitudes shape medical, scientific and public health problems, it will be difficult for us to deal with a problem as complex as AIDS in an effective and humane way.

Public Health and Social Disease

Barbara G. Rosenkrantz, Ph.D.
Professor, History of Science
Harvard University

When a public health need is identified, the decision to implement a corrective plan has only rarely been made soon after the need is felt. More often, a considerable time lag occurs and further delay in implementing any such plan is apparent. In the AIDS epidemic, scientific knowledge about the disease has increased rather dramatically in a very short period of time. An analysis of analogous historical perspectives may be useful in evaluating the selection of measures that are at our disposal to treat the present problem. It is not necessarily true, however, that this increase of public activity in these areas will be commensurate with the increase of scientific knowledge. Public understanding and concern about a disease has not very often resulted in public responsibility and action.

In the early 20th century in Massachusetts, there was considerable public interest in providing more publicly supported care for patients suffering from cancer. At this period of time, the diagnosis of and prognosis for patients with cancer was dismal, even more so than the current treatments and prognosis for patients with AIDS today. In the face of that kind of expectation and hope, the Massachusetts legislature directed the state public health department to aggressively provide publicly supported medical care for cancer patients. The public health department disagreed, arguing that it should not be in the position of providing care in a medical area where it lacked sufficiently sophisticated treatment or knowledge to effect a meaningful change. Thus, the ambiguity of the relationship between knowledge and public expectations and the willingness of public bodies to act has been a problem for many years.

The question of whether and in what manner the state or other public health departments can and should act in the area of social disease has been compounded by the ambiguity of the definition of a social disease. Many people consider a social disease ordinarily to be a sexually transmitted disease. Historically, a social disease has been any disease that has a major bearing on the health and welfare of the population. In terms of the numbers of individuals affected with AIDS, I think that we are confronting a "social disease." Tuberculosis is another example of a social disease in which the state has been and could be active in controlling disease transmission through public health measures.

Social diseases are not necessarily those diseases that are communicated directly by personal contact. Also, all diseases that are contagious have not been considered social diseases. Smallpox, for example, while dramatically contagious, has not been considered a social disease, even though it has deadly public health consequences. Thus, the critical question that appears to determine whether the state and public health departments will support victims of social diseases in those diseases that have a social impact relates, in fact, to the ambiguous relationship between the susceptibility of the public to the disease and the behavior patterns of individuals who engender that susceptibility. Public criticisms about these patterns inhibit public action in a variety of ways. We must think seriously about public criticism of the AIDS victims and its relation to the social responsibility that we feel to provide research monies, facilities, and support for individuals with this disease.

An important question raised in patients with tuberculosis was whether, by identifying the individuals who were contagious, this would assist the patient in appropriately modifying their behavior, in seeking treatment, and in giving them the information that they required and society required in order to support their medical needs. The debates in this area have been less clearly identified as supporting individuals who are sick than they have been in supporting those individuals who might be afflicted and who are not sick. The historical experience has been on the whole, in relation to tuberculosis in particular, that rather than having a state-wide program, a society-wide program which provided support for the sick and protection for those who were possibly endangered, we have primarily restricted the activities of the sick and not provided them with the types of support they needed. Therefore, we have failed to provide society with a morally responsible and socially responsible program that deals with the problems of its members. We have a history of public health activity that suggests a questionable commitment to the more vulnerable individuals who are most at risk because they are sick, and more affected by the public health risk (or the policy adopted) than the rest of society.

Individual perceptions and definitions of social disease and public health responsibility have given rise to any number of peculiar approaches to public health programs. We have emphasized control of the transmission of diseases but have neglected social responsibility to those who are sick. We have developed economically stringent and narrow programs that ignore social responsibility as a whole. The absence of support services for individuals with AIDS is an example of the narrow focus public programs tend to adopt. Separation of public health concerns into prevention, treatment, and research have resulted in patients falling through the cracks in each system, without any approach taking into account the entire spectrum of problems confronting the patient.

Perhaps one reason why research on prevention and research on treatment have been historically separated in the United States is that the legitimate realm of inquiry and activity for public health has been ordinarily restricted to the area of the prevention of transmission of disease rather than the treatment of individuals who are sick. This bifurcation between what we see as a united and associated situation has had seriously negative effects both on the sick and the well, supported by the notion that we have two separate health systems; one which deals with prevention and public health, and the other that deals with treatment and the health of those who can afford to stay healthy.

Funding for public health and prevention programs has generally been quite low. Consequently, the public health officials could only emphasize education and patience. That was the history of tuberculosis; it should not be seen as a template for public health response to all social disease. When we separate these considerations of prevention and treatment, it is a reflection, in part, not only of the manner in which we examine science and medicine but the manner in which our society views problems of social disease, education, and many other aspects of life which are part of modern society. The antituberculosis movement in the early 20th century encountered serious difficulties in providing the support that was needed to reduce the amount of disease because of these separate approaches. Those of us who are interested in the scientific aspects of disease control and those of us who are interested in the social aspects of disease control share a common concern. It is therefore desirable that the methods of funding research and support for prevention and treatment be organized in Congress, supported in our public agencies, and understood by our society as an entity, with the entire patient's health in mind.

Global Distribution of AIDS

Sheldon Landesman, M.D.
Associate Professor of Medicine
Downstate Medical Center, New York
Director, AIDS Study Group

In dealing with the AIDS problem in the United States, we tend to have less than a complete perspective of the disease. AIDS is not only a problem in the United States; it is clear that we are dealing with a pandemic. Throughout the world, the infection is slowly but steadily spreading to many other areas of the globe. At the present time, other than the United States, the area most severely affected by this pandemic is central Africa. In Rwanda, as many as 5% of the population tested may be antibody positive for HTLV-III. In some areas of Zaire, you may have also as many as 5% of the population test antibody positive. A significant amount of disease is present in both of these countries.

In addition, western Europe is facing problems similar to those we are facing here in this country. The incidence of AIDS in Paris and Geneva now rivals that of Los Angeles. There is reportedly no disease in eastern Europe. Apparently, the disease is illegal there.

It has become more evident that the patterns of spread of the disease in areas outside of the United States are, to some extent, different from the patterns or modes of transmission of the disease within the United States. In countries such as Zaire, Rwanda, and perhaps Haiti, the role of heterosexual transmission, the use of nonsterile needles, either for medicinal purposes or, on occasion, for scarification or tatooing, and blood transfusions may play a more significant role in the transmission of the disease. The disease has frightening implications in some of these countries because of the relative lack of sophistication of the medical community and/or their ancillary support staff. For example, in Haiti, nearly 40% of the women with AIDS had received a blood transfusion within four years of diagnosis of the disease.[7] It appears as though the blood transfusion was the principal mode of transmission for those particular women.

There are other broad implications of the epidemic outside of the immediate concerns of blood or sexual-borne transmission. We live in an era where global travel is very common. Governments here and abroad have begun to evaluate questions of who should or should not be allowed into a given area or a given country. If the virus continues to spread in Africa and, if at the same time, significant famine is present, many of the persons in these famine-stricken areas may migrate to other countries. Western Europe receives a significant number of these people who are leaving their famine-stricken countries. There is a host of geopolitical concerns that are beginning to surface. What steps will be taken in that area are not predictable. A worst case scenario is that the governments of western Europe and/or the United States will close their doors to persons from Africa or will demand serological screening before entry is allowed into the country. There is considerable precedent in this country to quarantine or to keep people out of this country on the basis of the presence of communicable or transmissible diseases. Similar policies are typical in many countries in Europe.

Countries elsewhere in the world are beginning to view the United States in the same manner that we are beginning to look at Africa. Knowledgeable and powerful voices may be heard, from Australia to France and to Germany, who suggest that the travel of Americans into these countries is one means of introducing the virus and that steps should be taken to restrict the travel of Americans. This obviously raises grave concerns about the civil liberties of the people involved and also has trade and economic implications. This epidemic is creating a subdued, yet clearly present, worldwide hysteria. At this time, we need to continue to think carefully about the issues, listen to each other, and continue to attempt to develop reasonable solutions.

Question

With respect to the presence of AIDS in central Africa, is there evidence as to how long the viral infection and the disease have been around, or where it (or they) came from? Many people believe that the gay population somehow invented a disease or are somehow being responsible for bringing it into this culture. Would it have happened under any circumstances?

Answer

There is a great deal of speculation and, unfortunately, very little evidence at the present time about the role of central Africa in this disease. It is absurd and unfortunate that the concept of gay people "inventing" the disease is prevalent. One has to be equally cautious in concluding that it is the Africans who "invented" the disease. The disease appears to be the result of a biological variation in a virus that in its present form has severe adverse consequences on the host it invades. The persons or the populations invaded are simply the unfortunate victims, not the originators of the virus or the disease. At the present time, there is significant disease in Zaire, especially in its capital, Kinshasa. The city has undergone an extremely rapid urbanization, from approximately 300,000 to 3,000,000 persons in the last 10 years. Whether the persons from the country brought the disease into the city is unclear. At the eastern end of Zaire, closer to central sub-Saharan Africa, a fair amount of faint seropositivity is found without disease expression. North of the eastern Zaire area is the country of Rwanda where there is a great deal of the disease; again, a high degree of seropositivity is found.

What has been suggested to explain these data is that perhaps the HTLV-III virus existed in a different form or type of virus which existed in the countryside in central Africa. Perhaps it infected many of the people there but, in fact, did not cause disease. Maybe it was a common virus indigenous to the area. This may explain why the eastern Zaire population has faint seropositivity without disease. Somewhere or somehow, the virus mutated into a more virulent form. Perhaps the first mutation occurred in the Zaire area adjacent to Rwanda. It then spread, through heterosexual transmission in the area of Rwanda and somehow was transported through travel into the western half of Zaire; eventually, through simply accident or fate, it arrived simultaneously in the United States and in Haiti. That is one scenario to explain its recent arrival; nobody knows for certain. Exactly where and how the virus was "born" is important and interesting, but presently unknown.

Comment

It has been typical for mankind to politicize disease. In previous centuries, syphilis was referred to as the "French disease" or the "Spanish curse," depending on your political perspective. It is an unfortunate, yet obviously a very human aspect of what we do in life to ascribe guilt or blame to members or groups in society that are really quite unwarranted.

Question

(Michael Callen): Dr. Landesman clearly believes that HTLV-III infection causes AIDS. I maintain that he presumes that AIDS is the same disease in each risk group, occurring in each risk group for the same reason at the same time via the same disease mechanism. According to the CDC criteria, a diagnosis of AIDS is one of exclusion. This is tantamount to suggesting that only one cause of immune deficiency remains to be discovered and that the cause of immune deficiency in a given patient is AIDS. To assume that what is occurring in Africa and what is occurring here, that the diseases are the same disease and that what links the different expressions of the disease is HTLV-III is a very tenuous assumption. It may be true; however, it may only be one link in a very long chain. There are other opinions as to why this disease is being expressed at this time that do not comport with your analysis.

Answer

Obviously, there are very important behavioral aspects to this disease. It is unfortunate, but as soon as we identify a behavioral component relating to a disease, we tend to focus on the behavioral cause, aspect, or expression to the exclusion of all others. For example, in cigarette smoking, because we know that smoking increases the risk of lung cancer, some people suggest that smokers should not be eligible for health insurance unless they stop smoking. Our society assumes that once we identify a behavior that puts a person at risk that person can alter the behavior. Behaviors are subject to social, cultural, political, personal, and psychological forces that often make them very difficult to change. To quit smoking is very difficult for many individuals. If we rely on the behavioral notion as a way of avoiding disease, we allow ourselves to be myopic about the disease. This is not to say that people who can make behavioral changes should not be encouraged to do so; it means only that to effect a behavioral change, the difficulties of altering behavior must be addressed. Society perpetuates the notion that some deaths are more poignant than others because some people have the behavioral ability to change and others do not. These gradations of empathy, based on notions of behavior—some people have control over their behavior, but some don't; therefore, some deaths are tragic and some aren't—are reprehensible. The loss of a life should not seem more or less clear because the person was, in part, responsible for his own demise. When the issue of behavior becomes inserted into a problem such as AIDS, it may have very powerful cultural and political implications.

Comment

It is possible that there may be other cofactors that could modify the expression of AIDS. It is not unique in the history of biology to have a large population infected with or exposed to, for example, the measles virus, yet only a certain small percentage of those exposed come down with the disease. More often than not, the cofactors responsible for resistance or susceptibility to the disease remain forever hidden somewhere in our genetic and immune composition. It would be a serious mistake to fail to acknowledge that the causative agent is HTLV-III; to do so would divert our energies away from the rapid development of a vaccine or agents to combat the viral infection. This is not a political, behavioral, or emotional issue. The virus is causing the disease. The rapid development of a vaccine or effective antiviral agent to prevent this disease is the single most important thing we can do at present.

References

1. Sontag, Susan. 1978. *Illness as metaphor.* New York: Random House.
2. Bulkey, L. Duncan. 1894. *Syphilis in the innocent.* New York.
3. What one woman has had to bear. 1912. *Forum* 48:451–453.
4. Kelly, Howard. 1906. The best way to treat the social evil. *Transactions of the American Society for Social and Moral Prophylaxis* 1:75.
5. Henig, Robin Marantz. 1983. AIDS: a new disease's deadly odyssey. *New York Times Magazine* (February 6):36.
6. See, for example, John Stokes. 1950. The practitioner and the antibiotic age of venereal disease control. *Venereal Disease Information* 31:13.
7. Pape, J.W., B. Liautaud, F. Thomas, et al. 1985. The acquired immunodeficiency syndrome in Haiti. *Annals of Internal Medicine* 103:674–678.

PART VIII
Issues In Social Science Research

Social Research On AIDS

Joan Sieber, Ph.D.
Professor of Psychology
California State University, Hayward

Much has been said about the various confidentiality-related concerns that arise in research on AIDS. Because these concerns are of overwhelming importance, it is easy to overlook more subtle ethical issues that arise when social scientists embark on AIDS research. I shall describe some aspects of a study of communication with persons at risk of AIDS as a context for pointing to the importance of some factors that affect the external validity of research on AIDS. Specifically, I shall point to the importance of (1) establishing continuing and sensitive lines of communication with the populations under study in order to keep abreast of the problems that become part of one's research, (2) bringing fresh social science insights to the problems of dealing with AIDS, and (3) continually testing psychological theory against the reality of AIDS-related problems so that the theory is tailored to the AIDS problem and not vice versa. Never before have social scientists undertaken to study such a kaleidoscopic phenomenon. The problems that we perceive to be connected with AIDS change with great rapidity, and in order to be effective, any program of research must be responsive to new information about the nature of the problem under study.

A wide range of conflicts, beliefs, fears, and mistrusts exist between and within the various communities that have an interest in addressing the problem of AIDS. The study of these attitudinal phenomena falls within the province of social science; for example, why does the straight community insist on regarding AIDS as a gay disease, a disease to which heterosexuals are invulnerable, a good topic for a dirty joke, and a topic one need not know much about? The AIDS virus may be spreading rapidly through the entire population while the straight community comforts itself with false beliefs of invulnerability. Why do some members of the gay community continue to expose themselves to extreme risk? What kinds of communication would result in more rational beliefs and behavior?

A pilot project is currently underway which addresses problems of communicating with persons about AIDS. A review of media coverage of AIDS during winter, 1985 revealed a great deal of information about the danger of AIDS to sexually active gay men. If indeed this media coverage was intended to induce high risk populations to take appropriate precautions, the assumption underlying the communication seemed to be that if one could sufficiently frighten persons at high risk of AIDS, they would limit themselves to safe sex or no sex.

Unfortunately, this is a wrong assumption. There is conclusive empirical evidence that the opposite is true: persons given fear-arousing warnings that do not describe effective means of coping with the threat are not likely to take appropriate precautions to avoid that threat. Rather, in response to fear arousing messages, persons continue to engage in self-destructive behavior precisely because it has become their response to anxiety and their means of temporarily reducing anxiety. Examples of such self-destructive behaviors include: overeating, smoking, alcohol and drug abuse, and risky sexual behavior. In the case of AIDS, public messages intended to encourage "safe sex" may contribute to a doomsday mentality for those who perceive it to be too late to change. Thus, as has often been reported in the gay community, an atmosphere of intense anxiety may increase, rather than decrease, promiscuous sexual activity. In effect, anonymous sex may lead both to anxiety about the disease and to lowered self-esteem, which, in turn, lead back to the same sexual behavior as a means of anxiety reduction.

Is this what is happening in the gay community? The rudimentary survey research literature currently available on AIDS indicates that whether a person engages in safe sex or reduces the number of their sexual partners is unrelated to level of education or level of information.[1] That is, telling an educated person a great deal about AIDS does not seem to produce more prudent behavior! Rather, the incidence of safe sex and of reducing number of sexual partners among gay men was greatest among those who had witnessed a person dying from AIDS.[1] How might these findings be explained?

There is a literature in social psychology on warning and "stress inoculation" which indicates that fear-arousing messages can be designed and delivered in such a way as to produce realistic assessment of risk and effective coping. Irving Janis[2] and his associates have shown that denial of danger and giving in to feelings of hopelessness are most characteristic of persons who have not been forced to take seriously the reality of the threat they face. Once persons acknowledge that awesome reality, they become amenable to a variety of procedures that enhance coping skills, provide courage and confidence, and promote feeling of hope and personal control. A variety of social psychological approaches have proven useful in instilling these qualities and producing effective coping behavior. To what extent are these psychological insights applied to AIDS patients?

I interviewed physicians who work with gay patients at risk of AIDS or who treat AIDS patients. I was told that the medical model of communication is entirely adequate for dealing with the problem. Physicians are always dealing with death and dying, and with people without hope of recovery. Essentially, there is nothing unusual about AIDS. The physicians I interviewed said that their patients were quite sophisticated and well-educated. The physicians tell their patients to have safe sex. The patients do not tell their physicians that they are not following orders, and thus the physicians conclude that their communications are effective. I am concerned that these physicians are wrong and that the medical community needs to inquire further into the efficacy of its mode of communication in this instance. The long incubation period, the stigma attached to AIDS, the fact that AIDS is, at this time, incurable, and that the diagnosis is not a clear-cut matter, all place AIDS in a very different category from other known infectious diseases.

How might physicians communicate more effectively with persons at risk of AIDS? My colleague Michael Patch and I have begun to evaluate the kinds of messages that might be designed to communicate with people at risk of AIDS. One of the things that Irving Janis and Leon Mann[3] have found to be most effective in enabling people to deal with a medical problem is to give them a sense of personal efficacy. The goal of my present research is to determine whether and how physicians might achieve this. Should this communication consist of advice about ways to strengthen the immune system, *e.g.*, by improving nutrition, getting lots of sleep, and reducing stress? What other elements should be added to increase a sense of personal efficacy and control, and to reduce denial or sense of hopelessness? Eventually, I expect to work with physicians in field experiments to determine the kinds of communication that are most effective in altering attitudes and behavior.

In some respects, our research can be modeled after that of Janis. In other respects, however, it raises a series of scientific and ethical problems that are new to social research on medical problems. When a social scientist seeks to study communication with, say, persons facing elective surgery, the problem the scientist sets out to study remains much the same over time. That is, the kinds of fears that surgery patients have do not change from month to month or year to year. However, the beliefs, attitudes, fears, mistrusts, concerns, and the sense of self-esteem that one has in relation to the disease AIDS probably varies within our culture on a week to week basis. Likewise, the knowledge and wisdom of the medical community is changing rapidly. The kinds of communication that would be ethical to experiment with depend on our current state of medical knowledge. How important are, say, sleep, nutrition, stress reduction, a support group, self-esteem, and feelings of personal efficacy? When does one risk providing false hope or a false sense of efficacy? What other social scientific theory can inform the way physicians and public health specialists communicate with persons at risk of AIDS? How can existing social theory be informed by and improved by a deeper understanding of AIDS patients, the surrounding culture, and the actual practices of physicians?

Validity is one of the hallmarks of ethical research. Externally valid social research on AIDS requires good theory that gives insight into the difficult social and psychological problems surrounding the disease. It also requires continual and sensitive monitoring and communication with all of the relevant communities to learn the emerging new parameters of the problem, and continual revision of one's theories and procedures to reflect the current state of knowledge and society.

Anxiety and Informed Consent

Barbara Stanley, Ph.D.
Chairperson, American Psychological Association Committee for
Protection of Human Participants in Research
Associate Professor, Department of Psychology, City University
of New York, John Jay College
Lecturer, Department of Psychiatry, Columbia University College
of Physicians and Surgeons

AIDS is a devastating illness that engenders enormous pain and suffering. For the physician who makes the diagnosis of AIDS and who conveys the diagnosis to patients, it is a very difficult, painful task. At some point, a physician must talk to the patient, describing the potential course and manifestations of the illness and the available treatment regimens, which vary with the different manifestations of the disease. The patient must be informed and decide whether to consent to whatever treatment is being proposed in a free and voluntary manner. The patient has an absolute right to refuse a medical procedure. Some patients do not want to have information about the illness. An area of concern to psychologists is the effect that giving information on morbidity has on the patient. This concern is not only a problem specific to patients with AIDS; in fact, there are no data that evaluate the informed consent process with AIDS patients. However, the empirical studies of patients who are afflicted with other diseases may be predictive about areas of concern in the informed consent process in AIDS patients.

A question that arises in the informed consent area is whether and to what degree does the medical information cause anxiety and stress. While the circumstance surrounding the disease causes a significant amount of stress, it does not appear as though more information causes more stress. Several studies have compared levels of anxiety in a given population of people with illness and the role of stress in the informed consent process.[4-7] Some of the people were given minimal information about their disease; other study participants were given a great deal of information about the disease and the recommended treatment. The anxiety was not any greater in participants given information than those who were not. In fact, there are studies that show that uncertainty may be more anxiety-provoking than knowledge, even if the news is bad news.[4] Thus, the axiom of withholding information in an effort to protect the patient from psychological harm or upset does not really seem to be the case. In certain instances, especially where it is ascertained that the information cannot be processed in a rational manner, withholding information may be a proper strategy for the psychological welfare of the patient. In general, however, patients do not become any more upset by receiving information. Some studies suggest that patients receive some degree of comfort in learning about their illness.[4] It seems then that the factors other than the level of information may contribute to a patient's anxiety. Of course, the knowledge itself that one is ill, can cause severe upset. But there are other factors that influence the psychological status of the patient. Included among these is the manner of presentation of the information to the patient, and the verbal and nonverbal attitudes of the physician conveying the information. It appears as though people want to receive relatively specific information about their illnesses and the risks associated with the proposed treatment, even if it seems as though it increases anxiety. Patients still want to know what fate has in store for them. One study compared what the physicians thought patients wanted to know about their disease and the available treatments; the patients consistently wanted more information and in much greater detail than the physicians thought they wanted. In light of these generic findings, it is not unreasonable to assume that patients with AIDS will be at least no more anxious, and possibly less so, by having complete medical information about their disease. By providing the information, we can assist, in at least one way, AIDS patients to begin to come to terms with their illness.

Sociomedical Research Priorities in AIDS

John L. Martin, Ph.D., M.P.H.
Division of Sociomedical Sciences
Columbia University School of Public Health

I direct an epidemiologic project at Columbia University that is focused on the social, psychological, and behavioral impact of the AIDS epidemic on healthy gay men. The study is a two-way panel study and has been supported by the National Institute of Mental Health for the past three years. We are beginning the field work aspects of interviewing 700 members of New York City's gay community who have decided to participate in the study. Each interview lasts several hours. In order to generate a sample size of 700 participants which adequately reflects the diversity of the urban gay population, my colleagues and I spent much time working with individuals and gay organizations in New York. It is impossible for a study such as this to maintain a low profile. I have had ample opportunity to solicit reactions to all aspects of the study from many segments of the community. Many of these reactions have been supportive, some have been neutral, while others have been hostile.

One specific hostile reaction to this study related to myself and the other principal investigators receiving large sums of money to study social, psychological, and behavioral changes in healthy men when unhealthy men afflicted with AIDS are dying every day. They argue that the only ethical course of action is to fund treatment, not sociomedical research. If there were a treatment for AIDS, then there would be no need for these studies of its impact. My initial reaction was to argue that less than 3% of all AIDS funding has gone to this sort of "psychosocial research." Further, the award has no relationship, competitive or otherwise, to funds allocated for biomedical research. In fact, the funding of this project represents serious recognition of the needs of the gay community insofar as that money could have been spent on other mental health research unrelated to AIDS or gay men.

As I thought about the criticism further, I realized my response, while accurate, was incomplete from the standpoint of our current need for answers to some basic and pressing sociomedical questions. Without a doubt, discovering effective therapies, developing a cure and a vaccine are of the highest priority in the long run. However, these goals, particularly a viable vaccine, are a number of years away. There is a large and growing population for whom the fruits of this research will simply be too late. What is needed now is an intensive educational campaign to inform people about effective but less elegant modes of prevention and control. The situation is analogous to John Snow stemming a cholera epidemic in London by removing the pump handle to the water pump, thereby preventing access to the contaminated water supply. Those people still needed water, however; alternative sources of sanitary water had to be found. In the AIDS area, I do not believe that we are in a position to conduct education to effect medically useful change based on data about social and sexual habits currently available. The information currently available is too nonspecific, too inconsistent, and too limited to expect the development of effective education programs and compliance on the scale now required.

There are three general areas of research which must be aggressively pursued if we intend to be effective in controlling AIDS in the near future. These areas require combining the substance and methods of both social science and biomedical science, which is a major challenge in itself.

The first area involves disease transmission factors. The importance of work in this area cannot be overstated since it forms the basis of broad public health policy and risk reduction guidelines. Unfortunately, the quality of research with respect to sexual behavior has been less than optimal both methodologically and substantively. We continue to lack instruments that reliably and validly measure the qualitative and quantitative aspects of sexual behavior. Questions regarding reliability and validity of self-reported sexual behavior are simply not addressed in medical and epidemiologic risk factor literature. As a result, what actually gets measured as sexual behavior tends to be idiosyncratic in study after study.

Furthermore, logical inconsistencies resulting from premature attempts to assign relative risk values to sex acts keep recurring. For example, in terms of contracting AIDS, passive anal intercourse rates as one of the riskiest sex acts for gay men. However, the active position in sexual relations with prostitutes is apparently what puts heterosexual men at risk for AIDS. More research is needed to determine the relative risk of each, and then, to convince the public to alter their respective sexual habits accordingly. It is likely that questions surrounding AIDS transmission by casual contact such as kissing will surface again as more comprehensive evidence is assembled regarding viral shedding. Right now, however, it is thought that kissing is considered to be a relatively safe sexual act in terms of viral transmission. It is practiced vigorously by people engaged in "safe sex," since casual contact is generally regarded as having low risk in AIDS transmission.

The main dilemma we must resolve is how to formulate public education efforts based on incomplete information. The public now looks to biomedical and sociomedical scientists to tell them how to conduct their sexual affairs. This reliance will increase as the AIDS epidemic grows. The least we can do is provide internally consistent information based on a standard set of sound measures while explicitly recognizing the limits of current knowledge.

The second area in need of combined efforts in biomedical and sociomedical science involves the establishment of risk gradients within currently identified at-risk groups. Not all gay men, IV drug users, or hemophiliacs are at equal risk of developing AIDS. However, there is a tendency to view these groups as virtually homogeneous with regard to illness risk. While labeling individuals at "high risk" based on group membership status may have been useful in the early stages of the epidemic, it would be far preferable, both medically and socially, to shift the emphasis towards describing the risk in terms of individual factors rather than group factors.

One such factor might be quantified by an index of prior known contact with persons with AIDS. That index would take into account duration, frequency, and type of contact. Such a measure deployed in large and diverse samples would provide some means of weighing the relative contribution of transmission factors as against host factors in illness expression. At this time we do not even know whether a lover of a person with AIDS is at significantly higher risk of developing illness compared with other gay men with and without lovers. Not only are we lacking information on risks associated with relatively simple individual characteristics, but there have not yet been any efforts expended to evaluate competing risks. Some of these questions could be answered with more comprehensive surveillance data.

Refocusing the definition risk towards individual factors and away from the relatively crude group membership status is useful not only for members of those risk groups, but also for others who do not choose to identify themselves as members of those groups, but who nevertheless belong by virtue of their behavior. Specifically, I am becoming increasingly aware of men who view themselves as "straight," who have families and suburban homes, yet regularly frequent bathhouses and tearooms for sex. Many of these men do not take appropriate precautions in these settings because they don't view themselves as being at risk for AIDS since they are not "gay." This is a dangerous state of affairs. If greater efforts were made to describe and publicize the risk factors for AIDS in more individual behavioral terms, more accurate assessments—both private and public—of everyone's risk would be possible.

The third area in need of combined efforts of biomedical and sociomedical scientists is in determining the relative importance of various cofactors in disease expression. Cofactors are other agents, substances, events, or conditions that are necessary or highly important in the development of illness given an etiologic agent. To the extent that the classic infectious disease model holds true for AIDS and cofactors indeed do play a significant role in AIDS illness, it means that some set of conditions that previously were benign may now be lethal in the presence of HTLV-III. For example, inhaled nitrates, a subclinical cytomegalovirus infection, or some other event normally resulting in a self-correcting immune imbalance may now lead to or promote the development of AIDS in the presence of HTLV-III.

Exactly what these cofactors are and the extent to which they can substitute for one another or act synergistically require research protocols that are biologically, socially, and behaviorally comprehensive. Research on cofactors may hold the most promise for reducing the incidence of AIDS in the next few years, given the apparently large and growing segments of the population that have evidence of prior HTLV-III exposure.

In conducting this research, the question of timing of cofactor events in relation to HTLV-III exposure is especially important to keep in mind. Although events occurring prior to or in conjunction with HTLV-III exposure may be important (*e.g* a significantly positive history of sexually transmitted diseases), it may also be possible that cofactor events occurring after HTLV-III exposure are most critical. This latter model might help explain the highly variable but often lengthy incubation period associated with AIDS. For those people who find they are positive to HTLV-III exposure it will be important for them to know whether future actions, over which they have control, will make a significant difference in developing AIDS. If the significant cofactor events lie in one's past, a different set of coping strategies may be required than if the significant cofactor events have yet to occur.

Although many of the ethical issues raised in these proceedings are the result of recently instituted, ongoing research, there is a number of ethical and social problems that we currently are confronted with because research that might bear on these issues has not been done. Answers to questions in the three areas I have outlined would not only be useful to compel people to take effective preventive measures but also would eliminate certain social and ethical problems we now face because we either lack answers or lack confidence in the answers we do have.

One last point summarizes one of the most difficult problems confronting all people having anything to do with AIDS, scientific or otherwise. AIDS is the leading cause of death among young men due to illness in New York and San Francisco. It is not a socially "respectable" cause of death. When famous men succumb in these cities to AIDS, the underlying cause of death listed in the newspapers is not AIDS. One reads only of a rare form of cancer, a pneumonia, or a battle with an unknown virus. The reasons for these euphemisms is to avoid public announcement of homosexuality. Since successful artists, designers, actors, writers, and scientists are rarely IV drug users, hemophiliacs, or Haitians, death due to AIDS can mean nothing else. In the public's eye, this illness is not just a marker for sexual preference, but indicates a promiscuous life lacking morals and restraint. So long as this prejudice and set of attributions prevail, suffering due to the threat of AIDS will ruin many fine lives. But few things in this world will be more painful than having the illness itself and trying to keep it a secret because of shame.

Issues in AIDS Epidemiology

William M. Hamilton, Ph.D.
Assistant State Epidemiologist for
the State of New Hampshire
AIDS Action Committee, Boston

While extraordinarily rapid progress has been made in many areas of AIDS research since 1981, the following crucial epidemiologic issues remain: first, the delineation of the natural history of AIDS and the AIDS-related complex (ARC); second, whether and to what extent the presence of antibodies to HTLV-III correlates with prognosis or with the ability to transmit the virus to others; and third, whether susceptibility to AIDS is mediated through or enhanced by environmental, behavioral, or host cofactors or by repeated exposure.

Answers to these questions will depend upon our ability to enroll patients and participants in large multicenter longitudinal studies. This ability, in turn, will depend upon the degree to which high risk groups are willing to participate. As others have pointed out, AIDS has resulted in a crisis in confidence with respect to those at risk. Most are well aware of the need for research subject participation in order to understand, treat, and prevent this truly devastating disease. And yet there is an understandable reluctance to provide information which potential subjects fear may be used against them. As researchers, we are in a particularly difficult and delicate position in that our study populations must be drawn in large part from already oppressed groups that are highly vulnerable to even greater social, political, and economic discrimination. Thus, to protect themselves from the possibility of still harsher social sanctions than those experienced to date, potential research subjects face the distressing choice of refusing to participate or providing inaccurate or incomplete data.

Our problem, then, is to develop data collection and record linkage procedures and policies which will both ensure maximum confidentiality as well as permit the rapid acquisition of large quantities of accurate and often extremely personal information. This is not an easy task, especially in that we must not only satisfy ourselves that a subject's privacy will be maintained. We must also convince and reassure the groups involved that this is being done and being done well. We are dealing here with the need to affirm simultaneously two basic ethical principles, namely, the respect for individuals as autonomous agents in control of their own destinies, and the pursuit of the common good of maximizing benefits and minimizing harms to both society and its individual elements. As researchers and as members of society we must unequivocally demonstrate our steadfast commitment to the principle that all persons are due a full and equal measure of compassion and respect. Without a clear public and unequivocal demonstration of that commitment, we risk failure both as scientists and as moral human beings.

Without reiterating the carefully developed guidelines for confidentiality in AIDS research from the Hastings Center, I have concentrated briefly on the particular areas where I see potential for conflict between the individual's right to privacy and the special needs of the epidemiologist.[8]

At the present time reporting of AIDS cases is mandatory in over 40 states. This incidence data, along with additional demographic, social, medical, and sexual information, is submitted to the Centers for Disease Control. Names are retained on state and local records but removed from data sent to the CDC. As yet, no formal surveillance programs of persons with AIDS-related conditions have been instituted, other than by the U.S. military, although with the widespread availability and use of the HTLV-III antibody test, more extensive surveillance of seropositive individuals may soon be undertaken.

It is of vital importance that we track the incidence rates over time, by geographic area, as well as by other demographic characteristics, in order to allocate properly available research and medical resources. Furthermore, since substantial but as yet unknown numbers of antibody positive individuals are known to be virus positive and theoretically capable of transmitting the virus, it is critical that we follow groups of antibody and virus positive persons over time to determine the natural history of these two states. Similarly, the long-term clinical implications of those with AIDS-related conditions are unknown. Only by follow-up over time can the utility of the antibody test and the ramifications of the AIDS-related clinical manifestations be assessed.

Such follow-up, however, requires repeated contacts with surveillance and research subjects which in turn requires the ability to identify and to locate these individuals. Herein lies the conflict between epidemiologic research needs and the individuals' rights to privacy and autonomy. In simple case enumeration activities and one-time cross sectional studies, personal identifiers can be removed from the data and destroyed, if necessary, once the diagnosis has been confirmed or the data abstraction form checked for accuracy and completeness.

Unfortunately, such assurances cannot be given to participants in longitudinal studies. There must, however, be substantive and convincing assurances of confidentiality. Otherwise, we cannot expect nor should we ask people to participate in research which carries with it such substantial risk of increased social oppression and extraordinarily severe personal hardship.

As Novick so succinctly stated, "The risk to each of these men and women would be that their voluntarily sharing the details of their private lives could easily be used against them with major social consequences. The risk to society is also massive in allowing the modern precedent of the violation of private lives as a reward for cooperation in important research."[9] It would be a Pyrrhic victory indeed for the biomedical research community to conquer AIDS only to find that in doing so we have broken and destroyed the very people we sought to save.

Question

Do you have any advice or comments on how researchers could develop access to funding sources for the kinds of social/biomedical research that you have described?

Answer

In Congress and in most health agencies of the government, social scientific research is an extremely low priority item. For example, the CDC decided to do a prospective study on hemophiliacs exposed to HTLV-III virus to determine who developed AIDS, who did not, and why not. A psychological study, designed to probe whether any psychoimmunological factors, family factors, or other factors had a relation to development of the disease, was dropped by the CDC as not being important. The only advice I can offer is to raise the issues with the CDC and with your congressman. Psychological, social science, and behavioral science research is inexpensive, very useful, and should be supported.

Question

Is anyone performing sociologic or psychologic research on the effects of AIDS in the gay population?

Answer

The National Institute of Mental Health has funded a very few studies in this area, although it is complicated by the lack of base data on the health or mental health of gay men. The funding had not been available prior to the AIDS crisis to perform the base data studies.

Comments

It is a possibility that social and psychological research may not have been done in the past because there may have been a fear that the outcomes could indicate that steps had to be taken at a different level than at the level of the people who get the disease. It is easy to discuss behavioral changes in "other people," such as gay men or IV drug abusers, who should change their behavior. If psychosocial research reveals that a relative lack of civil rights, positive self-esteem, and positive self-regard tend to encourage defensive, isolating, and now, potentially deadly behaviors, then the changes necessary to alter the behaviors include altering the attitudes and perceptions of people who contribute to these isolating tendencies. The attitudes of the status quo may contribute to the very behaviors that elicit, in some people, the disease. Some of this research may be too threatening.

References

1. McKusick, L., W. Hortsman, and T.J. Coates. 1985. AIDS and sexual behavior reported by gay men in San Francisco. *American Journal of Public Health* 75:493–496.
2. Janis, I.L. 1983. Stress inoculation in health care: Theory and research. In *Stress reduction and prevention,* ed. D. Meichenbaum and M.E. Jaremko. New York: Plenum Press.
3. Janis, I.L., and L. Mann. 1977. *Decision Making.* New York: Free Press.
4. Denney, M., D. Williamson, and R. Penn. 1975. Informed consent: emotional responses of patients. *Postgraduate Medicine* 60:205–209.
5. Lankton, J., B. Batchelder, and A. Onnislay. 1977. Emotional responses to detailed risk disclosure for anesthesia. *Anesthesiology* 46:294–296.
6. Houts, P., and D. Leaman. 1980. Patient responses to information about possible complications of medical procedures. Paper presented at the annual meeting of the American Psychological Association, September 1–5, Montreal, Canada.
7. Alfidi, R. 1971. Informed consent: a study of patient reaction. Journal of the American Medical Association 216:1325–1329.
8. Bayer, Ronald, Carol Levine, and Thomas H. Murray. 1984. Guidelines for confidentiality in research on AIDS. *IRB* 6(6):1–7.
9. Novick, Alvin. 1984. At risk for AIDS: confidentiality in research and surveillance. *IRB* 6(6):10–11.

Appendix
Ethical Issues in Psychological Research on AIDS

Committee for Protection of Human Participants in Research
in cooperation with the Committee on Gay Concerns
American Psychological Association*

Research that addresses quickly developing, highly publicized, and socially sensitive topics often raises acute ethical dilemmas. Current research on the psychological aspects of acquired immune deficiency syndrome (AIDS) offers an especially prominent and sensitive context for exploration of these ethical problems. The "usual" dilemma in deciding whether to conduct human research, of balancing potential social benefits against potential costs to individual participants, is starkly raised in research on AIDS. The groups at highest risk for AIDS (i.e., gay/bisexual men and intravenous drug users) are already liable in many jurisdictions for criminal penalties or social stigma. The process of investigation raises the spectre of exacerbation of these risks to participants. However, there is a great public interest in solving this public health problem. The public interest is obviously shared by AIDS patients, persons at risk for AIDS, and the "worried well" who perceive themselves at risk. Thus, potential participants may themselves have mixed interests, i.e., a desire to preserve anonymity and privacy, coupled with a profound wish for increased knowledge as to the etiology and treatment of AIDS. In the midst of such dilemmas, researchers are likely to encounter substantial pressure to "bend the rules" in regard, for example, to confidentiality of participants and premature disclosure of data.

Core Principles

The *Ethical Principles of Psychologists* provide some guidance to researchers involved in studies of AIDS. The psychologist's primary obligation is to "respect the dignity and worth of the individual and strive for the preservation and protection of fundamental human rights" (Preamble). Researchers must consider the welfare of participants (Preamble; Principle 6) and guard their civil rights (Principle 3c). This basic value on the integrity and worth of the individual is balanced by the responsibility to use professional skills to increase knowledge useful in the promotion of human welfare (Preamble; Principle 9).

It is quite possible that behavioral science can contribute significantly to an

---

understanding of the etiology of AIDS and amelioration of its consequences. Through examination of behaviors and psychological states of those members of at-risk groups who in fact contract the disease, psychological research might help to show the complex relationship between emotions and health, as well as between stress and immunosuppression. Such research might also illuminate the means of transmission of AIDS and, ultimately, ways of reducing the risk of contracting it. Psychologists may contribute to an understanding of ways to prevent or alleviate the distress experienced by people who have AIDS, their families and friends, persons in fact at risk, and persons who may perceive themselves erroneously to be at risk. Psychological research may also assist in understanding several aspects (e.g., neuropsychological involvement, psychoneuroimmunology) of the disease process itself.

In the midst of complex and sometimes competing public and individual interests, researchers bear an especially weighty obligation to consider carefully the relative risks and benefits of possible research on AIDS (Principles 1a, 9, 9a, 9b, and 9g). In deciding whether and how to conduct such studies, psychologists should deliberate personally and in consultation with peers and the public. In addition to use of standard procedures for consultation (e.g., consideration by an Institutional Review Board), it will very often be helpful to establish advisory groups drawn from the populations to be studied. Such extraordinary review serves several purposes. It increases the likelihood that proper attention is given to the various interests relevant to a decision as to whether and how a study is designed, implemented, and reported. It also provides protection of participants from "overresearch" and undue exploitation. Extraordinary review also serves as a check on the methodological integrity of the study, which is important for scientific purposes and to the determination of whether the study is sufficiently promising to warrant imposition upon participants and possible threats to their privacy. Research with gay men, for example, is less likely to result in ineffective recruitment of participants, failure to ask the most probative questions, or misinterpretation of data (and accompanying deleterious social consequences), if representatives of gay groups are consulted. However, it is important to note that consultation—even intensive consultation with peers and affected groups—does not absolve the researcher of ethical responsibility for the study and its conduct (Principle 9c), even when all legal requirements for review are met. On the other hand, careful ethical deliberation does not, of course, abrogate the requirement to follow legal procedures for protection of human participants (Principles 3d and 9). Especially when there is persistent pressure for answers to the public health issues, researchers need to remain ethically vigilant in all phases of the investigation. Each step in the study is likely to present its own risk/benefit calculus. (Note that principle 9 is organized more or less on parallel with the chronology of an investigation.)

Special Issues

Privacy

Respect for persons demands respect for the boundaries of the person—for preservation of a zone of privacy around personal information and bodily integrity. Psychological research on AIDS is difficult ethically in large part because of the intrusions upon individual privacy which result from the social interest in gaining knowledge relevant to the maintenance of public health.

Intrusiveness. Psychological research on AIDS is likely to have an intrusive quality because it involves inquiry into matters commonly considered intimate or sensitive. Research on risk factors and modes of transmission is apt to include questioning about participants' sexual practices, drug-taking history, past illnesses, relationships, history of travel, and other private matters. Questioning about one's feelings about AIDS, and even simply the express identification of participants as members of groups especially at risk for AIDS, may be stressful. Assessment of mental status may also be perceived as intrusive.

It is not just the content of the research protocols which is likely to be intrusive. Means of recruitment of participants may also raise questions of invasion of privacy. Examples include receiving a letter inviting participation with a return address on the envelope indicating the nature of the project, or being stopped by a researcher as one leaves a gay bar.

In general, researchers should minimize the unnecessary intrusiveness of their studies. Whenever possible, data should be derived from clinical interviews and archives which have already been collected. When practical, potential participants should be contacted only after they have volunteered directly, or permission for contact has been obtained by an appropriate intermediary who has identified the participant (e.g., personal physician; or the AIDS patient, when the population to be studied includes patients' lovers or acquaintances). When more intrusive procedures appear necessary for the conduct of a study, the researcher is especially obligated to consider and seek advice about the merits of the study in the face of the invasion of privacy (Principles 9 and 9a). The researcher should warn potential participants when the content of an interview or questionnaire may be disturbing (Principles 9d and 9f) and permit them to refrain from participating or to withdraw if they choose (Principle 9g). As discussed in more detail later in this statement, careful debriefing and follow-up should be undertaken to identify and prevent or alleviate stressful effects of participation (Principles 9g and 9i).

Principle 9f on its face prohibits *any* involuntary research. As indicated above, in virtually all cases this principle should be followed. However, there may be circumstances in which the state will exercise its police power to protect the public health and coerce the production of information which is believed necessary to understand and control the spread of AIDS. In such a circumstance, we are not prepared to say that psychologists should never participate in the design or implementation of legally sanctioned involuntary research (cf. Principle 3d). In fact, autonomy may already be substantially diminished in such an instance, and the additional data gathering may be a minimal intrusion justified by the principle of beneficence and the potential social good. It is important to emphasize, however, that the fact that a particular kind of research passes legal scrutiny does not absolve investigators of their obligation to consider the ethical calculus of the merits of the study. When participation is coerced, it is especially important to minimize intrusive questioning.

Confidentiality. Perhaps the most acute ethical problems in research on AIDS involve possible attempts to breach confidentiality. The protection of confidentiality is a "primary obligation" of psychologists (Principle 5; see also Principle 9j). This duty is based on several principles of ethics and social policy. First, the content of communications may be intimate, as in most psychological research on AIDS. Unintended exposure of these personal details is a serious intrusion on human dignity (cf. Preamble; Principle 9). Second, as already noted, respect for persons demands protection of individuals' autonomy in decision making about disclosure of private information. Third, there may be adverse consequences for the participants from the disclosure of information about behavior which may be subject to criminal penalties, financial difficulties (e.g., loss of employment, housing, and medical insurance), or at least social stigma. It is easy to imagine an industrious prosecutor using research files as a tool in a criminal investigation of homosexuals (whose sexual behavior may be prohibited by law) or drug users. Fourth, unintended disclosure of data may chill the public's willingness to participate in future research or researchers' willingness to conduct investigations on socially sensitive topics.

In fact, there have been some controversial releases of names of AIDS patients in the files of the Centers for Disease Control, which has already had a chilling effect on the collection and reporting of data. Moreover, as states require reporting of AIDS cases, the question arises of particularized disclosure of names or other identifying information through judicial or administrative subpoenas or the Freedom of Information Act.

Against the risk of breach of confidentiality, there are competing risks of *failing* to keep identifiable information. Longitudinal research and post hoc identification and investigation of subgroups which appear to be of special interest may be important in tracking the factors involved in the etiology of AIDS. Moreover, if certain patterns of factors, on the bases of future analyses, appear to be particularly important, participants may want to be locatable, especially if the information provides a means of diminishing the risk of contracting AIDS or increasing the success of treatment.

As a general rule, researchers should adopt methodological strategies (e.g., randomized response methods) and take legal steps (e.g., obtain protective orders or confidentiality certificates; promote legislative enactment of a researcher's privilege) before a study is conducted, in order to minimize the possibility of involuntary disclosure of data (Principles 1b, 3d, 5, 5a, 5b, 5c, and 9d). In some instances, confidentiality certificates which bar subpoena of data may be obtained from the Department of Health and Human Services. However, it is important to note that the scope of protection accorded by the certificates is unclear and has not been tested in the courts. For example, the statute authorizing the certificate simply bars subpoena of names or other identifying characteristics "which could lead directly or undirectly by reference to other information to identification of the research subjects." Therefore, a subpoena of the data given by a known participant may be enforceable. Also, researchers need to apply for the certificates in advance and they are not automatically granted.

In deciding whether to consent to participate, potential participants should be informed as to the limits of confidentiality and risks of unintended disclosure before consent to participate is given (Principles 5, 9d, and 9j). In cases where there is a desire to retain identifiable data, participants should be informed of the potential risks and benefits of doing so and given an option of having their data stored. Researchers should make diligent efforts to resist attempts to compel the disclosure of data (Principle 3d). Subpoenas, for example, may often be quashed or limited because of the public interest in the integrity of the research and the preservation of confidential relationships, or the lack of relevance or necessity for the evidence.

Debriefing and Follow-up

Because of the emotion-laden nature of the topic of AIDS, investigators should be careful to debrief participants and follow up appropriately (Principles 9g, 9h, and 9i). In some instances, the very knowledge that one is in a group which the investigator believes to have special significance for understanding AIDS may be traumatic. In other instances, in the course of a study, information may be obtained (e.g., whether an individual has HTLV-III antibodies) which may provide some indication of a participant's vulnerability to AIDS. In such circumstances, participants should be so informed. However, the precise meaning of the results of tests (such as the presence of HTLV-III antibodies) is often unknown or uncertain. It is presumptuous of investigators to withhold potentially bad news which may be important in future decisions by participants; it is obligatory in such instances to give *more* information, not less. Participants need to be made aware of the uncertainty or ambiguity in the meaning of particular findings. In providing such information, psychologists should use their own and their colleagues' information about ways of presenting information to maximize the probability that participants will have an accurate understanding of the results (for example, the application of base rates to a calculation of risk). Careful attention also should be given to participants' likely emotional responses to the information. Research on AIDS demands more than perfunctory counseling. The investigator should identify potential worries of participants and give information to allay or prevent undue concern before the individual makes a decision to participate. In debriefing, the researcher should discover what concerns remain (or were stimulated by the study) and take appropriate steps to alleviate them.

Reporting the Results

Just as there are special issues in reporting individual results to participants, there are also special considerations in the report of the study's findings to the broader community (see Principles 1a and 1c). The clamor for information on the etiology and treatment of AIDS is clear and understandable. The profound consequences of the illness, the uncertainty about it, and the stigma already attached to the groups at risk have combined to create an urgency—even panic—for rapid research and dissemination of findings. In that regard, the Assistant Secretary of Health and Human Services, Edward Brandt, took the unprecedented step of urging major journals to expedite review and publication of research on AIDS and to make prepublication announcements of relevant findings, once manuscripts had been approved by peer reviewers. Besides the public interest in quick acquisition and dissemination of scientific knowledge about AIDS, researchers may feel substantial self-interest in being first to report significant information about a "hot" topic.

Midst these pressures, it is important that researchers not lose sight of the social sensitivity of the topic. At a minimum, no service is done by reporting data for which conclusions cannot be obtained because the data have been inadequately analyzed or are based on an inadequate or skewed sample. Mistaken reports, even if well intended, can result in unwise public policy, public alarm (or undue complacency), and stigma for affected groups. When preliminary data suggest ways of reducing risk, there must be a determination of whether the potential benefits of the possibly valid warnings are outweighed by the harm which may result if the findings are ultimately determined to be erroneous. In a matter of great moment, there may be an imperative to facilitate research and its dissemination, but such an imperative is not furthered by abandonment of the principles of scientific investigation and communication.

Because of the significance which is likely to be attached to new findings about AIDS, it is especially incumbent upon investigators to report the limitations of their study and to emphasize points of uncertainty and alternative interpretations

(Principle 1a). In that regard, researchers should be careful to retain control over dissemination of the information insofar as possible (Principle 1c). Time might well be spent preparing news releases which explain the research, its import, and limitations in terms clearly understandable by policy makers and the public as a whole. Care should also be take to ensure that results cannot be interpreted in such a way as to blame AIDS patients for the condition they must endure (Principle 1a).

Suggestions for Further Reading

American Psychological Association. (1981). Ethical Principles of Psychologists. *American Psychologist*, 36, 633–638.

Batchelor, W.F. (ed.). (1984). AIDS [Section on Psychology in the Public Forum]. *American Psychologist*, 39, 1277–1314.

Boruch, R.F., & Cecil, J.S. (1979). *Methods of assuring confidentiality in social science research*. Philadelphia: University of Pennsylvania Press.

Council on Scientific Affairs, American Medical Association. (1984). The acquired immunodeficiency syndrome: Commentary. *Journal of the American Medical Association*, 252, 2037–2043. [A concise review of research and issues about AIDS.]

Knerr, C.R., Jr. (1982). What to do before and after a subpoena of data arrives. In J.E. Sieber (ed.), *The ethics of social research: Surveys and experiments* (pp. 191–206). New York: Springler-Verlag.

Marin, S.F., & Batchelor, W.F. (1984). Responding to the Psychological Crisis of AIDS. *Public Health Reports*, 99, 4–9.

Marwick, C. (1983). "Confidentiality" issues may cloud epidemiologic studies of AIDS. *Journal of American Medical Association*, 250, 1945–1946.

Nelson, R.L., & Hedrick, T.E. (1983). The statutory protection of confidential research data: Synthesis and evaluation. In F. Boruch & J.S. Cecil (eds.), *Solutions to ethical and legal problems in social research* (pp. 213–236). New York: Academic Press.

Pincus, H.A. (1984). AIDS, drug abuse, and mental health. *Public Health Reports*, 99, 106–108.

Zich, J., & Temoshok, L. (in press). A primer of pitfalls and opportunities in AIDS research. In D.A. Feldman (ed.), *AIDS and social science*. Unpublished manuscript.

PART IX
Guidelines for the Management of AIDS Patients

As more cases of AIDS are diagnosed, health care professionals in many settings are trying to institute AIDS infection control procedures in their facilities. The PRIM&R conference on which this book is based included several workshops that addressed AIDS infection control in practical terms. Since these workshops did not lend themselves to being transcribed and edited as were the preceding articles, this part attempts to recreate the useful, hands-on approach of the workshops. This part pools many resources that a health care professional can turn to in writing an AIDS policies and procedures manual.

In the first half are recommendations and precautions from the Centers for Disease Control's *Morbidity and Mortality Weekly Report*. The second half includes AIDS infection control procedures already adopted by several Boston-area facilities. Policies from several health care settings, including ambulance companies, home health agencies, and public hospitals, are represented.

It is a useful exercise to review the various CDC guidelines and see how different facilities incorporate these recommendations into policies and procedures that fit their professional and administrative needs. For example, consider the information that the CDC offers in response to the following questions that health care facilities may ask about AIDS: How do health care workers protect themselves and others from exposure to the AIDS virus? What precautions should be taken to keep the already immunosuppressed AIDS patient from coming in contact with new and potentially lethal infections? How can health care workers reduce the risk of subjecting AIDS patients to undue psychological and physical isolation in their efforts to stop the spread of the AIDS virus? Are certain health care workers, such as pregnant women, at greater risk in caring for AIDS patients? Are such employees justified in requesting to be excused from direct patient care? Based on the CDC guidelines, the policies and procedures presented below address these and many other concerns.

The Case Definition of AIDS

Centers for Disease Control

For the limited purposes of national reporting of some of the severe late manifestations of infection with human T-lymphotropic virus, type III/lymph-adenopathy-associated virus (HTLV-III/LAV) in the United States, CDC defines a case of "acquired immunodeficiency syndrome" (AIDS) as an illness characterized by:

I. one or more of the opportunistic diseases listed below (diagnosed by methods considered reliable) that are at least moderately indicative of underlying cellular immunodeficiency, and

II. absence of all known underlying causes of cellular immunodeficiency (other than HTLV-III/LAV infection) and absence of all other causes of reduced resistance reported to be associated with at least one of those opportunistic diseases.

Despite having the above, patients are excluded as AIDS cases if they have negative result(s) on testing for serum antibody to HTLV-III/LAV*, do not have a positive culture for HTLV-III/LAV, and have both a normal or high number of T-helper (OKI4 or LEU3) lymphocytes and a normal or high ratio of T-helper to T-suppressor (OKT8 or LEU2) lymphocytes. In the absence of test results, patients satisfying all other criteria in this definition are included as cases.

This general case definition may be made more explicit by specifying:

I. the particular diseases considered at least moderately indicative of cellular immunodeficiency, which are used as indicators of AIDS, and

II. the known causes of cellular immunodeficiency, or other causes of reduced resistance reported to be associated with particular diseases, which would disqualify a patient as an AIDS case.

This specification is as follows:

I. *Diseases at least moderately indicative of underlying cellular immunodeficiency:*

In the following list of diseases, the required diagnostic methods with positive results are shown in parentheses. "Microscopy" may include cytology.

A. *Protozoal and Helminthic Infections:*

1. Cryptosporidiosis, intestinal, causing diarrhea for over 1 month (on histology or stool microscopy)

2. *Pneumocystis carinii* pneumonia (on histology, or microscopy of a "touch" preparation, bronchial washings, or sputum)

3. Strongyloidosis, causing pneumonia, central nervous system infection, or infection disseminated beyond the gastrointestinal tract (on histology)

---

* A single negative test for HTLV-III/LAV may be applied here if it is an antibody test by ELISA, immunofluorescent, or Western Blot methods, because such tests are very sensitive. Viral cultures are less sensitive but more specific, and so may be relied on if positive but not if negative. If multiple antibody tests have inconsistent results, the result applied to the case definition should be that of the majority. A positive culture, however, would over-rule negative antibody tests.

4. Toxoplasmosis, causing infection in internal organs other than liver, spleen, or lymph nodes (on histology or microscopy of a "touch" preparation)

B. *Fungal Infections:*

1. Candidiasis, causing esophagitis (on histology, or microscopy of a "wet" preparation from the esophagus, or endoscopic or autopsy findings of white plaques on an erythematous mucosal base, but not by culture alone)

2. Cryptococcosis, causing central nervous system or other infection disseminated beyond lungs and lymph nodes (on culture, antigen detection, histology, or India ink preparation of CSF)

C. *Bacterial Infections:*

1. *Mycobacterium avium* or *intracellulare (Mycobacterium avium* complex), or *Mycobacterium kansasii,* causing infection disseminated beyond lungs and lymph nodes (on culture)

D. *Viral Infections:*

1. Cytomegalovirus, causing infection in internal organs other than liver, spleen, or lymph nodes (on histology or cytology, but not by culture or serum antibody titer)

2. Herpes simplex virus, causing chronic mucocutaneous infection with ulcers persisting more than 1 month, or pulmonary, gastrointestinal tract (beyond mouth, throat, or rectum), or disseminated infection (but not encephalitis alone) (on culture, histology, or cytology)

3. Progressive multifocal leukoencephalopathy (presumed to be caused by Papovavirus) (on histology)

E. *Cancer:*

1. Kaposi's sarcoma (on histology)

2. Lymphoma limited to the brain (on histology)

F. *Other Opportunistic Infections with Positive test for HTLV-III/LAV*:*

In the absence of the above opportunistic diseases, any of the following diseases is considered indicative of AIDS if the patient had a positive test for HTLV-III/LAV*:

---

* A positive test for HTLV-III/LAV may consist of a reactive test for antibody to HTLV-III/LAV or a positive culture (isolation of HTLV-III/LAV from a culture of the patient's peripheral blood lympho-

1. disseminated histoplasmosis (on culture, histology, or cytology)

2. bronchial or pulmonary candidiasis (on microscopy or visualization grossly of characteristic white plaques on the bronchial mucosa, but not by culture alone)

3. isosporiasis, causing chronic diarrhea (over 1 month), (on histology or stool microscopy)

G. *Chronic lymphoid interstitial pneumonitis:*

In the absence of the above opportunistic diseases, a histologically confirmed diagnosis of chronic (persisting over 2 months) lymphoid interstitial pneumonisis in a child (under 13 years of age) is indicative of AIDS unless test(s) for HTLV-III/LAV are negative.* The histologic examination of lung tissue must show diffuse interstitial and peribronchiolar infiltration by lymphocytes, plasma cells with Russell bodies, plasmacytoid lymphocytes and immunoblasts. Histologic and culture evaluation must not identify a pathogenic organism as the cause of this pneumonia.

H. *Non-Hodgkin's Lymphoma with Positive Test for HTLV-III/LAV*:*

If the patient had a positive test for HTLV-III/LAV*, then the following histologic types of lymphoma are indicative of AIDS, regardless of anatomic site:

1. Small *non*cleaved lymphoma (Burkitt's tumor or Burkitt-like lymphoma), but not small cleaved lymphoma,

2. Immunoblastic sarcoma (or immunoblastic lymphoma) of B-cell or unknown immunologic phenotype (not of T-cell type). Other terms which may be equivalent include: diffuse undifferentiated non-Hodgkin's lymphoma, large cell lymphoma (cleaved or noncleaved), diffuse histiocytic lymphoma, reticulum cell sarcoma, and high-grade lymphoma.

Lymphomas should not be accepted as indicative of AIDS if they are described in any of the following ways: low grade, of T-cell type (immunologic phenotype), small cleaved lymphoma, lymphocyte lymphoma (regardless of whether well or poorly differentiated), lymphoblastic lymphoma, plasmacytoid lymphocytic lymphoma, lymphocytic leukemia (acute or chronic), or Hodgkin's disease (or Hodgkin's lymphoma).

---

cytes). If multiple antibody tests have inconsistent results, the result applied to the case definition, should be that of the majority done by the ELISA, immunofluorescent, or Western Blot methods. A positive culture, however, would over-rule negative antibody tests.

II. Known Causes of Reduced Resistance Known causes of reduced resistance to diseases indicative of immunodeficiency are listed in the left column, while the diseases that may be attributable to these causes (rather than to the immunodeficiency caused by HTLV-III/LAV infection) are listed on the right:

Known Causes of Reduced Resistance	Diseases Possibly Attributable to the Known Causes of Reduced Resistance
1. Systematic corticosteroid therapy	Any infection diagnosed during or within 1 month after discontinuation of the corticosteroid therapy, unless symptoms specific for an infected anatomic site (e.g., dyspnea for pneumonia, headache for encephalitis, diarrhea for colitis) began before the corticosteroid therapy
	or any cancer diagnosed during or within 1 month after discontinuation of more than 4 months of long-term corticosteroid therapy, unless symptoms specific for the anatomic sites of the cancer (as described above) began before the long-term corticosteroid therapy
2. Other immunosuppressive or cytotoxic therapy	Any infection diagnosed during or within 1 year after discontinuation of the immunosuppressive therapy, unless symptoms specific for an infected anatomic site (as described above) began before the therapy
	or any cancer diagnosed during or within 1 year after discontinuation of more than 4 months of long-term immunosuppressive therapy, unless symptoms specific for the anatomic sites of the cancer (as described above) began before the long-term therapy
3. Cancer of lymphoreticular or histiocytic tissue such as lymphoma (except for lymphoma localized to the brain), Hodgkin's disease, lymphocytic leukemia, or multiple myeloma	Any infection or cancer, if diagnosed after or within 3 months before the diagnosis of the cancer of lymphoreticular or histiocytic tissue
4. Age 60 years or older at diagnosis	Kaposi's sarcoma, but not if the patient has a positive test for HTLV-III/LAV
5. Age under 26 days (neonatal) at diagnosis	Toxoplasmosis or herpes simplex virus infection, as described above
6. Age under 6 months at diagnosis	Cytomegalovirus infection, as described above
7. An immunodeficiency atypical of AIDS, such as one involving hypogammaglobulinemia or angioimmunoblastic lymphadenopathy; or an immunodeficiency of which the cause appears to be a genetic or developmental defect, rather than HTLV-III/LAV infection	Any infection or cancer diagnosed during such immunodeficiency
8. Exogenous malnutrition (starvation due to food deprivation, not malnutrition due to malabsorption or illness)	Any infection or cancer diagnosed during or within 1 month after discontinuation of starvation

Recommendations for Preventing Transmission of Infection with Human T-Lymphotropic Virus Type III/ Lymphadenopathy-Associated Virus in the Workplace

Centers for Disease Control*

Persons at increased risk of acquiring infection with human T-lymphotropic virus type III/lymphadenopathy-associated virus (HTLV-III/LAV), the virus that causes acquired immunodeficiency syndrome (AIDS), include homosexual and bisexual men, intravenous (IV) drug abusers, persons transfused with contaminated blood or blood products, heterosexual contacts of persons with HTLV-III/ LAV infection, and children born to infected mothers. HTLV-III/LAV is transmitted through sexual contact, parenteral exposure to infected blood or blood components, and perinatal transmission from mother to neonate. HTLV-III/LAV has been isolated from blood, semen, saliva, tears, breast milk, and urine and is likely to be isolated from some other body fluids, secretions, and excretions, but epidemiologic evidence has implicated only blood and semen in transmission. Studies of nonsexual household contacts of AIDS patients indicate that casual contact with saliva and tears does not result in transmission of infection. Spread of infection to household contacts of infected persons has not been detected when the household contacts have not been sex partners or have not been infants of infected mothers. The kind of nonsexual person-to-person contact that generally occurs among workers and clients or consumers in the workplace does not pose a risk for transmission of HTLV-III/LAV.

As in the development of any such recommendations, the paramount consideration is the protection of the public's health. The following recommendations have been developed for all workers, particularly workers in occupations in which exposure might occur to blood from individuals infected with HTLV-III/ LAV. These recommendations reinforce and supplement the specific recommendations that were published earlier for clinical and laboratory staffs[1] and for dental-care personnel and persons performing necropsies and morticians' services.[2] Because of public concern about the purported risk of transmission of HTLV-III/LAV by persons providing personal services and by food and beverages, these recommendations contain information and recommendations for personal-service and food-service workers. Finally, these recommendations address workplaces in general where there is no known risk of transmission of HTLV-III/ LAV (e.g., offices, schools, factories, construction sites). Formulation of specific recommendations for health-care workers (HCWs) who perform invasive

---

* Reprinted from the *Morbidity and Mortality Weekly Report* 34(45):682–695 (November 15, 1985).

procedures (e.g., surgeons, dentists) is in progress. Separate recommendations are also being developed to prevent HTLV-III/LAV transmission in prisons, other correctional facilities, and institutions housing individuals who may exhibit uncontrollable behavior (e.g., custodial institutions) and in the perinatal setting. In addition, separate recommendations have already been developed for children in schools and day-care centers.[3]

HTLV-III/LAV-infected individuals include those with AIDS;[4] those diagnosed by their physician(s) as having other illnesses due to infection with HTLV-III/LAV; and those who have virologic or serologic evidence of infection with HTLV-III/LAV but who are not ill.

These recommendations are based on the well-documented modes of HTLV-III/LAV transmission identified in epidemiologic studies and on comparison with the hepatitis B experience. Other recommendations are based on the hepatitis B model of transmission.

Comparison with the Hepatitis B Virus Experience

The epidemiology of HTLV-III/LAV infection is similar to that of hepatitis B virus (HBV) infection, and much that has been learned over the last 15 years related to the risk of acquiring hepatitis B in the workplace can be applied to understanding the risk of HTLV-III/LAV transmission in the health-care and other occupational settings. Both viruses are transmitted through sexual contact, parenteral exposure to contaminated blood or blood products, and perinatal transmission from infected mothers to their offspring. Thus, some of the same major groups at high risk for HBV infection (e.g., homosexual men, IV drug abusers, persons with hemophilia, infants born to infected mothers) are also the groups at highest risk for HTLV-III/LAV infection. Neither HBV nor HTLV-III/LAV has been shown to be transmitted by casual contact in the workplace, contaminated food or water, or airborne or fecal-oral routes.[5]

HBV infection is an occupational risk for HCWs, but this risk is related to degree of contact with blood or contaminated needles. HCWs who do not have contact with blood or needles contaminated with blood are not at risk for acquiring HBV infection in the workplace.[6–8]

In the health-care setting, HBV transmission has not been documented between hospitalized patients, except in hemodialysis units, where blood contamination of the environment has been extensive or where HBV-positive blood from one patient has been transferred to another patient through contamination of instruments. Evidence of HBV transmission from HCWs to patients has been rare and limited to situations in which the HCWs exhibited high concentrations of virus in their blood (at least 100,000,000 infectious virus particles per ml of serum), and the HCWs sustained a puncture wound while performing traumatic procedures on patients or had exudative or weeping lesions that allowed virus to contaminate instruments or open wounds of patients.[9-11]

Current evidence indicates that, despite epidemiologic similarities of HBV and HTLV-III/LAV infection, the risk for HBV transmission in health-care settings far exceeds that for HTLV-III/LAV transmission. The risk of acquiring HBV infection following a needlestick from an HBV carrier ranges from 6% to 30%,[12,13] far in excess of the risk of HTLV-III/LAV infection following a needlestick involving a source patient infected with HTLV-III/LAV, which is less than 1%. In addition, all HCWs who have been shown to transmit HBV infection in health-care settings have belonged to the subset of chronic HBV carriers who, when tested, have exhibited evidence of exceptionally high concentrations of virus (at least 100,000,000 infectious virus particles per ml) in their blood. Chronic carriers who have substantially lower concentrations of virus in their blood have not been implicated in transmission in the health-care setting.[9-11,14] The HBV model thus represents a "worst case" condition in regard to transmission in health-care and other related settings. Therefore, recommendations for the control of HBV infection should, if followed, also effectively prevent spread of HTLV-III/LAV. Whether additional measures are indicated for those HCWs who perform invasive procedures will be addressed in the recommendations currently being developed.

Routine screening of all patients or HCWs for evidence of HBV infection has never been recommended. Control of HBV transmission in the health-care setting has emphasized the implementation of recommendations for the appropriate handling of blood, other body fluids, and items soiled with blood or other body fluids.

Transmission from Patients to Health-Care Workers

HCWs include, but are not limited to, nurses, physicians, dentists and other dental workers, optometrists, podiatrists, chiropractors, laboratory and blood bank technologists and technicians, phlebotomists, dialysis personnel, paramedics, emergency medical technicians, medical examiners, morticians, housekeepers, laundry workers, and others whose work involves contact with patients, their blood or other body fluids, or corpses.

Recommendations for HCWs emphasize precautions appropriate for preventing transmission of bloodborne infectious diseases, including HTLV-III/LAV and HBV infections. Thus, these precautions should be enforced routinely, as should other standard infection-control precautions, regardless of whether HCWs or patients are known to be infected with HTLV-III/LAV or HBV. In addition to being informed of these precautions, all HCWs, including students and housestaff, should be educated regarding the epidemiology, modes of transmission, and prevention of HTLV-III/LAV infection.

Risk of HCWs acquiring HTLV-III/LAV in the workplace

Using the HBV model, the highest risk for transmission of HTLV-III/LAV in the workplace would involve parenteral exposure to a needle or other sharp instrument contaminated with blood of an infected patient. The risk to HCWs of acquiring HTLV-III/LAV infection in the workplace has been evaluated in several studies. In five separate studies, a total of 1,498 HCWs have been tested for antibody to HTLV-III/LAV. In these studies, 666 (44.5%) of the HCWs had direct parenteral (needlestick or cut) or mucous membrane exposure to patients with AIDS or HTLV-III/LAV infection. Most of these exposures were to blood rather than to other body fluids. None of the HCWs whose initial serologic tests were negative developed subsequent evidence of HTLV-III/LAV infection following their exposures. Twenty-six HCWs in these five studies were seropositive when first tested; all but three of these persons belonged to groups recognized to be at increased risk for AIDS.[15] Since one was tested anonymously, epidemiologic information was available on only two of these three seropositive HCWs. Although these two HCWs were reported as probable occupationally related HTLV-III/LAV infection,[15,16] neither had a preexposure nor an early postexposure serum sample available to help determine the onset of infection. One case reported from England describes a nurse who seroconverted following an accidental parenteral exposure to a needle contaminated with blood from an AIDS patient.[17]

In spite of the extremely low risk of transmission of HTLV-III/LAV infection, even when needlestick injuries occur, more emphasis must be given to precautions targeted to prevent needlestick injuries in HCWs caring for any patient since such injuries continue to occur even during the care of patients who are known to be infected with HTLV-III/LAV.

Precautions to prevent acquisition of HTLV-III/LAV infection by HCWs in the workplace

These precautions represent prudent practices that apply to preventing transmission of HTLV-III/LAV and other bloodborne infections and should be used routinely.[18]

1. Sharp items (needles, scalpel blades, and other sharp instruments) should be considered as potentially infective and be handled with extraordinary care to prevent accidental injuries.

2. Disposable syringes and needles, scalpel blades, and other sharp items should be placed into puncture-resistant containers located as close as practical to the area in which they were used. To prevent needlestick injuries, needles should not be recapped, purposefully bent, broken, removed from disposable syringes, or otherwise manipulated by hand.

3. When the possibility of exposure to blood or other body fluids exist, routinely recommended precautions should be followed. The anticipated exposure may require gloves alone, as in handling items soiled with blood or equipment contaminated with blood or other body fluids, or may also require gowns, masks, and eye-coverings when performing procedures involving more extensive contact with blood or potentially infective body fluids, as in some dental or endoscopic procedures or postmortem examinations. Hands should be washed thoroughly and immediately if they accidentally become contaminated with blood.

4. To minimize the need for emergency mouth-to-mouth resuscitation, mouth pieces, resuscitation bags, or other ventilation devices should be strategically located and available for use in areas where the need for resuscitation is predictable.

5. Pregnant HCWs are not known to be at greater risk of contracting HTLV-III/LAV infections than HCWs who are not pregnant; however, if a HCW develops HTLV-III/LAV infection during pregnancy, the infant is at increased risk of infection resulting from perinatal transmission. Because of this risk, pregnant HCWs should be especially familiar with precautions for preventing HTLV-III/LAV transmission.[19]

Precautions for HCWs during home care of persons infected with HTLV-III/LAV

Persons infected with HTLV-III/LAV can be safely cared for in home environments. Studies of family members of patients infected with HTLV-III/LAV have found no evidence of HTLV-III/LAV transmission to adults who were not sexual contacts of the infected patients or to children who were not at risk for perinatal transmission.[3] HCWs providing home care face the same risk of transmission of infection as HCWs in hospitals and other health-care settings, especially if there are needlesticks or other parenteral or mucous membrane exposures to blood or other body fluids.

When providing health-care service in the home to persons infected with HTLV-III/LAV, measures similar to those used in hospitals are appropriate. As in the hospital, needles should not be recapped, purposefully bent, broken, removed from disposable syringes, or otherwise manipulated by hand. Needles and other sharp items should be placed into puncture-resistant containers and disposed of in accordance with local regulations for solid waste. Blood and other body fluids can be flushed down the toilet. Other items for disposal that are contaminated with blood or other body fluids that cannot be flushed down the toilet should be wrapped securely in a plastic bag that is impervious and sturdy (not easily penetrated). It should be placed in a second bag before being discarded in a manner consistent with local regulations for solid waste disposal. Spills of blood or other body fluids should be cleaned with soap and water or a household detergent. As in the hospital, individuals cleaning up such spills should wear disposable gloves. A disinfectant solution or a freshly prepared solution of sodium hypochlorite (household bleach, see below) should be used to wipe the area after cleaning.

Precautions for providers of prehospital emergency health care

Providers of prehospital emergency health care include the following: paramedics, emergency medical technicians, law enforcement personnel, firefighters, lifeguards, and others whose job might require them to provide first-response medical care. The risk of transmission of infection, including HTLV-III/LAV infection, from infected persons to providers of prehospital emergency health care should be no higher than that for HCWs providing emergency care in the hospital if appropriate precautions are taken to prevent exposure to blood or other body fluids.

Providers of prehospital emergency health care should follow the precautions outlined above for other HCWs. No transmission of HBV infection during mouth-to-mouth resuscitation has been documented. However, because of the theoretical risk of salivary transmission of HTLV-III/LAV during mouth-to-mouth resuscitation, special attention should be given to the use of disposable airway equipment or resuscitation bags and the wearing of gloves when in contact with blood or other body fluids. Resuscitation equipment and devices known or suspected to be contaminated with blood or other body fluids should be used once and disposed of or be thoroughly cleaned and disinfected after each use.

Management of parenteral and mucous membrane exposures of HCWs

If a HCW has a parenteral (e.g., needlestick or cut) or mucous membrane (e.g., splash to the eye or mouth) exposure to blood or other body fluids, the source patient should be assessed clinically and epidemiologically to determine the likelihood of HTLV-III/LAV infection. If the assessment suggests that infection may exist, the patient should be informed of the incident and requested to consent to serologic testing for evidence of HTLV-III/LAV infection. If the source patient has AIDS or other evidence of HTLV-III/LAV infection, declines testing, or has a positive test, the HCW should be evaluated clinically and serologically for evidence of HTLV-III/LAV infection as soon as possible after the exposure, and, if seronegative, retested after 6 weeks and on a periodic basis thereafter (e.g., 3, 6, and 12 months following exposure) to determine if transmission has occurred. During this follow-up period, especially the first 6–12 weeks, when most infected persons are expected to seroconvert, exposed HCWs should receive counseling about the risk of infection and follow U.S. Public Health Service (PHS) recommendations for preventing transmission of AIDS.[20,21] If the source patient is seronegative and has no other evidence of HTLV-III/LAV infection, no further follow-up of the HCW is necessary. If the source patient cannot be identified, decisions regarding appropriate follow-up should be individualized based on the type of exposure and the likelihood that the source patient was infected.

Serologic testing of patients

Routine serologic testing of all patients for antibody to HTLV-III/LAV is not recommended to prevent transmission of HTLV-III/LAV infection in the workplace. Results of such testing are unlikely to further reduce the risk of transmission, which, even with documented needlesticks, is already extremely low. Furthermore, the risk of needlestick and other parenteral exposures could be reduced by emphasizing and more consistently implementing routinely recommended infection-control precautions (e.g., not recapping needles). Moreover, results of routine serologic testing would not be available for emergency cases and patients with short lengths of stay, and additional tests to determine whether a positive test was a true or false positive would be required in populations with a low prevalence of infection. However, this recommendation is based only on considerations of occupational risks and should not be construed as a recommendation against other uses of the serologic test, such as for diagnosis or to facilitate medical management of patients. Since the experience with infected patients varies substantially among hospitals (75% of all AIDS cases have been reported by only 280 of the more than 6,000 acute-care hospitals in the United States), some hospitals in certain geographic areas may deem it appropriate to initiate serologic testing of patients.

Transmission From Health-Care Workers to Patients

Risk of transmission of HTLV-III/LAV infection from HCWs to patients

Although there is no evidence that HCWs infected with HTLV-III/LAV have transmitted infection to patients, a risk of transmission of HTLV-III/LAV infection from HCWs to patients would exist in situations where there is both (1) a high degree of trauma to the patient that would provide a portal of entry for the virus (e.g., during invasive procedures) and (2) access of blood or serous fluid from the infected HCW to the open tissue of a patient, as could occur if the HCW sustains a needlestick or scalpel injury during an invasive procedure. HCWs known to be infected with HTLV-III/LAV who do not perform invasive procedures need not be restricted from work unless they have evidence of other infection or illness for which any HCW should be restricted. Whether additional restrictions are indicated for HCWs who perform invasive procedures is currently being considered.

Precautions to prevent transmission of HTLV-III/LAV infection from HCWs to patients

These precautions apply to all HCWs, regardless of whether they perform invasive procedures: (1) All HCWs should wear gloves for direct contact with mucous membranes or nonintact skin of all patients and (2) HCWs who have exudative lesions or weeping dermatitis should refrain from all direct patient care and from handling patient-care equipment until the condition resolves.

Management of parenteral and mucous membrane exposures of patients

If a patient has a parenteral or mucous membrane exposure to blood or other body fluids of a HCW, the patient should be informed of the incident and the same procedure outlined above for exposures of HCWs to patients should be followed for both the source HCW and the potentially exposed patient. Management of this type of exposure will be addressed in more detail in the recommendations for HCWs who perform invasive procedures.

Serologic testing of HCWs

Routine serologic testing of HCWs who do not perform invasive procedures (including providers of home and prehospital emergency care) is not recommended to prevent transmission of HTLV-III/LAV infection. The risk of transmission is extremely low and can be further minimized when routinely recommended infection-control precautions are followed. However, serologic testing should be available to HCWs who may wish to know their HTLV-III/LAV infection status. Whether indications exist for serologic testing of HCWs who perform invasive procedures is currently being considered.

Risk of occupational acquisition of other infectious diseases by HCWs infected with HTLV-III/LAV

HCWs who are known to be infected with HTLV-III/LAV and who have defective immune systems are at increased risk of acquiring or experiencing serious complications of other infectious diseases. Of particular concern is the risk of severe infection following exposure to patients with infectious diseases that are easily transmitted if appropriate precautions are not taken (e.g., tuberculosis). HCWs infected with HTLV-III/LAV should be counseled about the potential risk associated with taking care of patients with transmissible infections and should continue to follow existing recommendations for infection control to minimize their risk of exposure to other infectious agents.[18,19] The HCWs' personal physician(s), in conjunction with their institutions' personnel health services or medical directors, should determine on an individual basis whether the infected HCWs can adequately and safely perform patient-care duties and suggest changes in work assignments, if indicated. In making this determination, recommendations of the Immunization Practices Advisory Committee and institutional policies concerning requirements for vaccinating HCWs with live-virus vaccines should also be considered.

Sterilization, Disinfection, Housekeeping, and Waste Disposal to Prevent Transmission of HTLV-III/LAV

Sterilization and disinfection procedures currently recommended for use [22,23] in health-care and dental facilities are adequate to sterilize or disinfect instruments, devices, or other items contaminated with the blood or other body fluids from individuals infected with HTLV-III/LAV. Instruments or other nondisposable items that enter normally sterile tissue or the vascular system or through which blood flows should be sterilized before reuse. Surgical instruments used on all patients should be decontaminated after use rather than just rinsed with water. Decontamination can be accomplished by machine or by hand cleaning by trained personnel wearing appropriate protective attire [24] and using appropriate chemical germicides. Instruments or other nondisposable items that touch intact mucous membranes should receive high-level disinfection.

Several liquid chemical germicides commonly used in laboratories and health-care facilities have been shown to kill HTLV-III/LAV at concentrations much lower than are used in practice.[25] When decontaminating instruments or medical devices, chemical germicides that are registered with and approved by the U.S. Environmental Protection Agency (EPA) as "sterilants" can be used either for sterilization or for high-level disinfection depending on contact time; germicides that are approved for use as "hospital disinfectants" and are mycobactericidal when used at appropriate dilutions can also be used for high-level disinfection of devices and instruments. Germicides that are mycobactericidal are preferred because mycobacteria represent one of the most resistant groups of microorganisms; therefore, germicides that are effective against mycobacteria are also effective against other bacterial and viral pathogens. When chemical germicides are used, instruments or devices to be sterilized or disinfected should be thoroughly cleaned before exposure to the germicide, and the manufacturer's instructions for use of the germicide should be followed.

Laundry and dishwashing cycles commonly used in hospitals are adequate to decontaminate linens, dishes, glassware, and utensils. When cleaning environmental surfaces, housekeeping procedures commonly used in hospitals are adequate; surfaces exposed to blood and body fluids should be cleaned with a detergent followed by decontamination using an EPA-approved hospital disinfectant that is mycobactericidal. Individuals cleaning up such spills should wear disposable gloves. Information on specific label claims of commercial germicides can be obtained by writing to the Disinfectants Branch, Office of Pesticides, Environmental Protection Agency, 401 M Street, S.W., Washington, D.C., 20460.

In addition to hospital disinfectants, a freshly prepared solution of sodium hypochlorite (household bleach) is an inexpensive and very effective germicide.[25] Concentrations ranging from 5,000 ppm (a 1:10 dilution of household bleach) to 500 ppm (a 1:100 dilution) sodium hypochlorite are effective, depending on the amount of organic material (e.g., blood, mucus, etc.) present on the surface to be cleaned and disinfected.

Sharp items should be considered as potentially infective and should be handled and disposed of with extraordinary care to prevent accidental injuries. Other potentially infective waste should be contained and transported in clearly identified impervious plastic bags. If the outside of the bag is contaminated with blood or other body fluids, a second outer bag should be used. Recommended practices for disposal of infective waste [23] are adequate for disposal of waste contaminated by HTLV-III/LAV. Blood and other body fluids may be carefully poured down a drain connected to a sanitary sewer.

Considerations Relevant to Other Workers

Personal-service workers (PSWs)

PSWs are defined as individuals whose occupations involve close personal contact with clients (e.g., hairdressers, barbers, estheticians, cosmetologists, manicurists, pedicurists, massage therapists). PSWs whose services (tattooing, ear piercing, acupuncture, etc.) require needles or other instruments that penetrate the skin should follow precautions indicated for HCWs. Although there is no evidence of transmission of HTLV-III/LAV from clients to PSWs, from PSWs to clients, or between clients of PSWs, a risk of transmission would exist from PSWs to clients and vice versa in situations where there is both (1) trauma to one of the individuals that would provide a portal of entry for the virus and (2) access of blood or serous fluid from one infected person to the open tissue of the other, as could occur if either sustained a cut. A risk of transmission from client to client exists when instruments contaminated with blood are not sterilized or disinfected between clients. However, HBV transmission has been documented only rarely in acupuncture, ear piercing, and tattoo establishments and never in other personal-service settings, indicating that any risk for HTLV-III/LAV transmission in personal-service settings must be extremely low.

All PSWs should be educated about transmission of bloodborne infections, including HTLV-III/LAV and HBV. Such education should emphasize principles of good hygiene, antisepsis, and disinfection. This education can be accomplished by national or state professional organizations, with assistance from state and local health departments, using lectures at meetings or self-instructional materials. Licensure requirements should include evidence of such education. Instruments that are intended to penetrate the skin (e.g., tattooing and acupuncture needles, ear piercing devices) should be used once and disposed of or be thoroughly cleaned and sterilized after each use using procedures recommended for use in health-care institutions. Instruments not intended to penetrate the skin but which may become contaminated with blood (e.g., razors), should be used for only one client and be disposed of or thoroughly cleaned and disinfected after use using procedures recommended for use in health-care institutions. Any PSW with exudative lesions or weeping dermatitis, regardless of HTLV-III/LAV infection status, should refrain from direct contact with clients until the condition resolves. PSWs known to be infected with HTLV-III/LAV need not be restricted from work unless they have evidence of other infections or illnesses for which any PSW should also be restricted.

Routine serologic testing of PSWs for antibody to HTLV-III/LAV is not recommended to prevent transmission from PSWs to clients.

Food-service workers (FSWs)

FSWs are defined as individuals whose occupations involve the preparation or serving of food or beverages (e.g., cooks, caterers, servers, waiters, bartenders, airline attendants). All epidemiologic and laboratory evidence indicates that bloodborne and sexually transmitted infections are not transmitted during the preparation or serving of food or beverages, and no instances of HBV or HTLV-III/LAV transmission have been documented in this setting.

All FSWs should follow recommended standards and practices of good personal hygiene and food sanitation.[26] All FSWs should exercise care to avoid injury to hands when preparing food. Should such an injury occur, both aesthetic and sanitary considerations would dictate that food contaminated with blood be discarded. FSWs known to be infected with HTLV-III/LAV need not be restricted from work unless they have evidence of other infection or illness for which any FSW should also be restricted.

Routine serologic testing of FSWs for antibody to HTLV-III/LAV is not recommended to prevent disease transmission from FSWs to consumers.

Other workers sharing the same work environment

No known risk of transmission to co-workers, clients, or consumers exists from HTLV-III/LAV-infected workers in other settings (e.g., offices, schools, factories, construction sites). This infection is spread by sexual contact with infected persons, injection of contaminated blood or blood products, and by perinatal transmission. Workers known to be infected with HTLV-III/LAV should not be restricted from work solely based on this finding. Moreover, they should not be restricted from using telephones, office equipment, toilets, showers, eating facilities, and water fountains. Equipment contaminated with blood or other body fluids of any worker, regardless of HTLV-III/LAV infection status, should be cleaned with soap and water or a detergent. A disinfectant solution or a fresh solution of sodium hypochlorite (household bleach, see above) should be used to wipe the area after cleaning.

Other Issues in the Workplace

The information and recommendations contained in this document do not address all the potential issues that may have to be considered when making specific employment decisions for persons with HTLV-III/LAV infection. The diagnosis of HTLV-III/LAV infection may evoke unwarranted fear and suspicion in some co-workers. Other issues that may be considered include the need for confidentiality, applicable federal, state, or local laws governing occupational safety and health, civil rights of employees, workers' compensation laws, provisions of collective bargaining agreements, confidentiality of medical records, informed consent, employee and patient privacy rights, and employee right-to-know statutes.

Development of These Recommendations

The information and recommendations contained in these recommendations were developed and compiled by CDC and other PHS agencies in consultation with individuals representing various organizations. The following organizations were represented: Association of State and Territorial Health Officials, Conference of State and Territorial Epidemiologists, Association of State and Territorial Public Health Laboratory Directors, National Association of County Health Officials, American Hospital Association, United States Conference of Local Health Officers, Association for Practitioners in Infection Control, Society of Hospital Epidemiologists of America, American Dental Association, American Medical Association, American Nurses' Association, American Association of Medical Colleges, American Association of Dental Schools, National Institutes of Health, Food and Drug Administration, Food Research Institute, National Restaurant Association, National Hairdressers and Cosmetologists Association, National Gay Task Force, National Funeral Directors and Morticians Association, American Association of Physicians for Human Rights, and National Association of Emergency Medical Technicians. The consultants also included a labor union representative, an attorney, a corporate medical director, and a pathologist. However, these recommendations may not reflect the views of individual consultants or the organizations they represented.

References

1. CDC. Acquired immune deficiency syndrome (AIDS): precautions for clinical and laboratory staffs. MMWR 1982;31:577-80.
2. CDC. Acquired immunodeficiency syndrome (AIDS): precautions for health-care workers and allied professionals. MMWR 1983;32:450-1.
3. CDC. Education and foster care of children infected with human T-lymphotropic virus type III/ lymphadenopathy-associated virus. MMWR 1985;34:517-21.
4. CDC. Revision of the case definition of acquired immunodeficiency syndrome for national reporting— United States. MMWR 1985;34:373-5.
5. CDC. ACIP recommendations for protection against viral hepatitis. MMWR 1985;34:313-24, 329-335.
6. Hadler SC, Doto IL, Maynard JE, et

al. Occupational risk of hepatitis B infection in hospital workers. Infect Control 1985;6:24–31.

7. Dienstag JL, Ryan DM. Occupational exposure to hepatitis B virus in hospital personnel: infection or immunization? Am J Epidemiol 1982; 115:26–39.

8. Pattison CP, Maynard JE, Berquist KR, et al. Epidemiology of hepatitis B in hospital personnel. Am J Epidemiol 1975;101:59–64.

9. Kane MA, Lettau LA. Transmission of HBV from dental personnel to patients. JADA 1985;110:634–6.

10. Hadler SC, Sorley DL, Acree KH, et al. An outbreak of hepatitis B in a dental practice. Ann Intern Med 1981;95:133–8.

11. Carl M, Blakey DL, Francis DP, Maynard JE. Interruption of hepatitis B transmission by modification of a gynaecologist's surgical technique. Lancet 1982;1:731–3.

12. Seeff LB, Wright EC, Zimmerman HJ, et al. Type B hepatitis after needlestick exposure: prevention with hepatitis B immune globulin. Ann Intern Med 1978;88:285–93.

13. Grady GF, Lee VA, Prince AM, et al. Hepatitis B immune globulin for accidental exposures among medical personnel: Final report of a multicenter controlled trial. J Infect Dis 1978;138:625–38.

14. Shikata T, Karasawa T, Abe K, et al. Hepatitis B e antigen and infectivity of hepatitis B virus. J Infect Dis 1977;136:571–6.

15. CDC. Update: evaluation of human T-lymphotropic virus type III/lymphadenopathy-associated virus infection in health-care personnel— United States. MMWR 1985;34: 575–8.

16. Weiss SH, Saxinger WC, Rechtman D, et al. HTLV-III infection among health care workers: association with needle-stick injuries. JAMA 1985;254:2089–93.

17. Anonymous. Needlestick transmission of HTLV-III from a patient infected in Africa. Lancet 1984;ii:1376–7.

18. Garner JS, Simmons BP. Guideline for isolation precautions in hospitals. Infect Control 1983;4:245–325.

19. Williams WW. Guideline for infection control in hospital personnel. Infect Control 1983;4:326–49.

20. CDC. Prevention of acquired immune deficiency syndrome (AIDS): report of inter-agency recommendations. MMWR 1983;32:101–3.

21. CDC. Provisional Public Health Service inter-agency recommendations for screening donated blood and plasma for antibody to the virus causing acquired immunodeficiency syndrome. MMWR 1985; 34:1–5.

22. Favero MS. Sterilization, disinfection, and antisepsis in the hospital. In: Manual of Clinical Microbiology. 4th ed. Washington, D.C.: American Society for Microbiology, 1985;129–37.

23. Garner JS, Favero MS. Guideline for handwashing and hospital environmental control, 1985. Atlanta Georgia: Centers for Disease Control, 1985. Publication no. 99-1117.

24. Kneedler JA, Dodge GH. Perioperative patient care. Boston: Blackwell Scientific Publications, 1983: 210–1.

25. Martin LS, McDougal JS, Loskoski SL. Disinfection and inactivation of the human T-lymphotropic virus type III/lymphadenopathy-associated virus. J Infect Dis 1985;152: 400–3.

26. Food Service Sanitation Manual 1976. DHEW publication no. (FDA) 78-2081. First printing June 1978.

Acquired Immune Deficiency Syndrome (AIDS): Precautions for Clinical and Laboratory Staffs

Centers for Disease Control*

The etiology of the underlying immune deficiencies seen in AIDS cases in unknown. One hypothesis consistent with current observations is that a transmissible agent may be involved. If so, transmission of the agent would appear most commonly to require intimate, direct contact involving mucosal surfaces, such as sexual contact among homosexual males, or through parenteral spread, such as occurs among intravenous drug abusers and possibly hemophilia patients using Factor VIII products. Airborne spread and interpersonal spread through casual contact do not seem likely. These patterns resemble the distribution of disease and modes of spread of hepatitis B virus, and hepatitis B virus infections occur very frequently among AIDS cases.

There is presently no evidence of AIDS transmission to hospital personnel from contact with affected patients or clinical specimens. Because of concern about a possible transmissible agent, however, interim suggestions are appropriate to guide patient-care and laboratory personnel, including those whose work involves experimental animals. At present, it appears prudent for hospital personnel to use the same precautions when caring for patients with AIDS as those used for patients with hepatitis B virus infection, in which blood and body fluids likely to have been contaminated with blood are considered infective. Specifically, patient-care and laboratory personnel should take precautions to avoid direct contact of skin and mucous membranes with blood, blood products, excretions, secretions, and tissues of persons judged likely to have AIDS. The following precautions do not specifically address out-patient care, dental care, surgery, necropsy, or hemodialysis of AIDS patients. In general, procedures appropriate for patients known to be infected with hepatitis B virus are advised, and blood and organs of AIDS patients should not be donated.

The precautions that follow are advised for persons and specimens from persons with: opportunistic infections that are not associated with underlying immunosuppressive disease or therapy; Kaposi's sarcoma (patients under 60 years of age); chronic generalized lymphadenopathy, unexplained weight loss and/or prolonged unexplained fever in persons who belong to groups with apparently increased risks of AIDS (homosexual males, intravenous drug abusers, Haitian entrants, hemophiliacs); and possible AIDS (hospitalized for evaluation). Hospitals and laboratories should adapt the following suggested precautions to their individual circumstances; these recommendations are not meant to restrict hospitals from implementing additional precautions.

---

*Reprinted from the *Morbidity and Mortality Weekly Report* 31(43):577–580 (November 5, 1982).

A. The following precautions are advised in providing care to AIDS patients:

1. Extraordinary care must be taken to avoid accidental wounds from sharp instruments contaminated with potentially infectious material and to avoid contact of open skin lesions with material from AIDS patients.

2. Gloves should be worn when handling blood specimens, blood-soiled items, body fluids, excretions, and secretions, as well as surfaces, materials, and objects exposed to them.

3. Gowns should be worn when clothing may be soiled with body fluids, blood, secretions, or excretions.

4. Hands should be washed after removing gowns and gloves and before leaving the rooms of known or suspected AIDS patients. Hands should also be washed thoroughly and immediately if they become contaminated with blood.

5. Blood and other specimens should be labeled prominently with a special warning, such as "Blood Precautions" or "AIDS Precautions." If the outside of the specimen container is visibly contaminated with blood, it should be cleaned with a disinfectant (such as a 1:10 dilution of 5.25% sodium hypochlorite [household bleach] with water). All blood specimens should be placed in a second container, such as an impervious bag, for transport. The container or bag should be examined carefully for leaks or cracks.

6. Blood spills should be cleaned up promptly with a disinfectant solution, such as sodium hypochlorite (see above).

7. Articles soiled with blood should be placed in an impervious bag prominently labeled "AIDS Precautions" or "Blood Precautions" before being sent for reprocessing or disposal. Alternatively, such contaminated items may be placed in plastic bags of a particular color designated solely for disposal of infectious wastes by the hospital. Disposable items should be incinerated or disposed of in accord with the hospital's policies for disposal of infectious wastes. Reusable items should be reprocessed in accord with hospital policies for hepatitis B virus-contaminated items. Lensed instruments should be sterilized after use on AIDS patients.

8. Needles should not be bent after use, but should be promptly placed in a puncture-resistant container used solely for such disposal. Needles should not be reinserted into their original sheaths before being discarded into the container, since this is a common cause of needle injury.

9. Disposable syringes and needles are preferred. Only needle-locking syringes or one-piece needle-syringe units should be used to aspirate fluids from patients, so that collected fluid can be safely discharged through the needle, if desired. If reusable syringes are employed, they should be decontaminated before reprocessing.

10. A private room is indicated for patients who are too ill to use good hygiene, such as those with profuse diarrhea, fecal incontinence, or altered behavior secondary to central nervous system infections.

Precautions appropriate for particular infections that concurrently occur in AIDS patients should be added to the above, if needed.

B. The following precautions are advised for persons performing laboratory tests or studies on clinical specimens or other potentially infectious materials (such as inoculated tissue cultures, embryonated eggs, animal tissues, etc.) from known or suspected AIDS cases:

1. Mechanical pipetting devices should be used for the manipulation of all liquids in the laboratory. Mouth pipetting should not be allowed.

2. Needles and syringes should be handled as stipulated in Section A (above).

3. Laboratory coats, gowns, or uniforms should be worn while working with potentially infectious materials and should be discarded appropriately before leaving the laboratory.

4. Gloves should be worn to avoid skin contact with blood, specimens containing blood, blood-soiled items, body fluids, excretions, and secretions, as well as surfaces, materials, and objects exposed to them.

5. All procedures and manipulations of potentially infectious material should be performed carefully to minimize the creation of droplets and aerosols.

6. Biological safety cabinets (Class I or II) and other primary containment devices (e.g., centrifuge safety cups) are advised whenever procedures are conducted that have a high potential for creating aerosols or infectious droplets. These include centrifuging, blending, sonicating, vigorous mixing, and harvesting infected tissues from animals or embryonated eggs. Fluorescent activated cell sorters generate droplets that could potentially result in infectious aerosols. Translucent plastic shielding between the droplet-collecting area and the equipment operator should be used to reduce the presently uncertain magnitude of this risk. Primary containment devices are also used in handling materials that might contain concentrated infectious agents or organisms in greater quantities than expected in clinical specimens.

7. Laboratory work surfaces should be decontaminated with a disinfectant, such as sodium hypochlorite solution (see A5 above), following any spill of potentially infectious material and at the completion of work activities.

8. All potentially contaminated materials used in laboratory tests should be decontaminated, preferably by autoclaving, before disposal or reprocessing.

9. All personnel should wash their hands following completion of laboratory activities, removal of protective clothing, and before leaving the laboratory.

C. The following additional precautions are advised for studies involving experimental animals inoculated with tissues or other potentially infectious materials from individuals with known or suspected AIDS.

1. Laboratory coats, gowns, or uniforms should be worn by personnel entering rooms housing inoculated animals. Certain nonhuman primates, such as chimpanzees, are prone to throw excreta and to spit at attendants; personnel attending inoculated animals should wear molded surgical masks and goggles or other equipment sufficient to prevent potentially infective droplets from reaching the mucosal surfaces of their mouths, nares, and eyes. In addition, when handled, other animals may disturb excreta in their bedding. Therefore, the above precautions should be taken when handling them.

2. Personnel should wear gloves for all activities involving direct contact with experimental animals and their bedding and cages. Such manipulations should be performed carefully to minimize the creation of aerosols and droplets.

3. Necropsy of experimental animals should be conducted by personnel wearing gowns and gloves. If procedures generating aerosols are performed, masks and goggles should be worn.

4. Extraordinary care must be taken to avoid accidental sticks or cuts with sharp instruments contaminated with body fluids or tissues of experimental animals inoculated with material from AIDS patients.

5. Animal cages should be decontaminated, preferably by autoclaving, before they are cleaned and washed.

6. Only needle-locking syringes or one-piece needle-syringe units should be used to inject potentially infectious fluids into experimental animals.

The above precautions are intended to apply to both clinical and research laboratories. Biological safety cabinets and other safety equipment may not be generally available in clinical laboratories. Assistance should be sought from a microbiology laboratory, as needed, to assure containment facilities are adequate to permit laboratory tests to be conducted safely.

Reported by Hospital Infections Program, Div of Viral Diseases, Div of Host Factors, Div of Hepatitis and Viral Enteritis, AIDS Activity, Center for Infectious Diseases, Office of Biosafety, CDC; Div of Safety, National Institutes of Health.

Acquired Immunodeficiency Syndrome (AIDS):
Precautions for Health-Care Workers
and Allied Professionals
Centers for Disease Control*

Acquired immunodeficiency syndrome (AIDS) was first recognized in 1981. The epidemiology of AIDS is consistent with the hypothesis that it is caused by a transmissible infectious agent.[1-3] AIDS appears to be transmitted by intimate sexual contact or by percutaneous inoculation of blood or blood products. There has been no evidence of transmission by casual contact or airborne spread, nor have there been cases of AIDS in health-care or laboratory personnel that can be definitely ascribed to specific occupational exposures.[4]

CDC has published recommended precautions for clinical and laboratory personnel who work with AIDS patients.[5] Precautions for these and allied professionals are designed to minimize the risk of mucosal or parenteral exposure to potentially infective materials. Such exposure can occur during direct patient care or while working with clinical or laboratory specimens and from inadvertent or unknowing exposure to equipment, such as needles, contaminated with potentially infective materials. Caution should be exercised in handling secretions or excretions, particularly blood and body fluids, from the following: (1) patients who meet the existing surveillance definition of AIDS;[1] (2) patients with chronic, generalized lymphadenopathy, unexplained weight loss, and/or prolonged unexplained fever when the patient's history suggests an epidemiologic risk for AIDS;[1,2] and (3) all hospitalized patients with possible AIDS.

These principles for preventing AIDS transmission also need to be adopted by allied professionals not specifically addressed in the previous publications but whose work may bring them into contact with potentially infective material from patients with the illnesses described in the above three groups.

---

*Reprinted from the *Morbidity and Mortality Weekly Report* 32(34):450–451 (September 2, 1983).

The following precautions are recommended for those who provide dental care, perform postmortem examinations, and perform work as morticians when working with persons with histories of illnesses described in the above three groups:

Dental-Care Personnel

1. Personnel should wear gloves, masks, and protective eyewear when performing dental or oral surgical procedures.
2. Instruments used in the mouths of patients should be sterilized after use.[5-9]

Persons Performing Necropsies or Providing Morticians' Services

1. As part of immediate postmortem care, deceased persons should be identified as belonging to one of the above three groups, and that identification should remain with the body.
2. The procedures followed before, during, and after the postmortem examination are similar to those for hepatitis B. All personnel involved in performing an autopsy should wear double gloves, masks, protective eyewear, gowns, waterproof aprons, and waterproof shoe coverings. Instruments and surfaces contaminated during the postmortem examination should be handled as potentially infective items.[5-7]
3. Morticians should evaluate specific procedures used in providing mortuary care and take appropriate precautions to prevent the parenteral or mucous-membrane exposure of personnel to body fluids.

These and earlier recommendations outline good infection control and laboratory practices and are similar to the recommendations for prevention of hepatitis B. As new information becomes available on the cause and transmission of AIDS, these precautions will be revised as necessary.

Reported by AIDS Activity, Div of Host Factors, Div of Viral Diseases, Hospital Infections Program, Center for Infectious Diseases, Office of Biosafety, CDC

References

1. CDC. Update on acquired immune deficiency syndrome (AIDS)—United States. MMWR 1982;31:507-8, 513-4.
2. Jaffe HW, Choi K, Thomas PA, et al. National case-control study of Kaposi's sarcoma and "*Pneumocystis carinii* pneumonia in homosexual men: Part 1, epidemiologic results. Ann Intern Med 1983;99:145-51.
3. Francis DP, Curran JW, Essex M. Epidemic acquired immune deficiency syndrome: Epidemiologic evidence for a transmissible agent. (guest editorial) JNCI 1983;71:1-4.
4. CDC. An evaluation of acquired immunodeficiency syndrome (AIDS) reported in health-care personnel—United States. MMWR 1983;32: 358-60.
5. CDC. Acquired immune deficiency syndrome (AIDS): precautions for clinical and laboratory staffs. MMWR 1982;31:577-80.
6. Simmons BP, with Hooton TM, Mallison GF. Guidelines for hospital environmental control. Infect Control 1981;2:131-46.
7. CDC guidelines on infection control. Guidelines for hospital environmental control (continued). Infect Control 1982;3:52-60.
8. Garner JS, Simmons BP. CDC-guideline for isolation precautions in hospitals. Infect Control 1983;4: 245-325.
9. Cooley RL, Lubow RM. AIDS: an occupational hazard? J Am Dent Assoc 1983;107:28-31.

Recommendations for Preventing Possible Transmission of Human T-Lymphotropic Virus Type III/ Lymphadenopathy-Associated Virus from Tears

Centers for Disease Control*

Human T-lymphotropic virus type III/lymphadenopathy-associated virus (HTLV-III/LAV), the etiologic agent of acquired immunodeficiency syndrome (AIDS), has been found in various body fluids, including blood, semen, and saliva. Recently, scientists at the National Institutes of Health isolated the virus from the tears of an AIDS patient.[1] The patient, a 33-year-old-woman with a history of *Pneumocystis carinii* pneumonia and disseminated *Mycobacterium avium-intracellulare* infection, had no ocular complaints, and her eye examination was normal. Of the tear samples obtained from six other patients with AIDS or related conditions, three showed equivocal culture results, and three were culture-negative.

The following precautions are judged suitable to prevent spread of HTLV-III/ LAV and other microbial pathogens that might be present in tears. They do not

---

*Reprinted from the *Morbidity and Mortality Weekly Report* 34(34):533-534 (August 30, 1985).

apply to the procedures used by individuals in caring for their own lenses, since the concern is the possible virus transmission between individuals.

1. Health-care professionals performing eye examinations or other procedures involving contact with tears should wash their hands immediately after a procedure and between patients. Handwashing alone should be sufficient, but when practical and convenient, disposable gloves may be worn. The use of gloves is advisable when there are cuts, scratches, or dermatologic lesions on the hands. Use of other protective measures, such as masks, goggles or gowns, is *not* indicated.

2. Instruments that come into direct contact with external surfaces of the eye should be wiped clean and then disinfected by: (a) a 5- to 10-minute exposure to a fresh solution of 3% hydrogen peroxide; or (b) a fresh solution containing 5,000 parts per million (mg/L) free available chlorine—a 1/10 dilution of common household bleach (sodium hypochlorite); or (c) 70% ethanol; or (d) 70% isopropanol. The device should be thoroughly rinsed in tap water and dried before reuse.

3. Contact lenses used in trial fittings should be disinfected between each fitting by one of the following regimens:
   a. Disinfection of trial hard lenses with a commercially available hydrogen peroxide contact lens disinfecting system currently approved for soft contact lenses. (Other hydrogen peroxide preparations may contain preservatives that could discolor the lenses.) Alternatively, most trial hard lenses can be treated with the standard heat disinfection regimen used for soft lenses (78–80 C [172–176 F] for 10 minutes). Practitioners should check with hard lens suppliers to ascertain which lenses can be safely heat-treated.
   b. Rigid gas permeable (RGP) trial fitting lenses can be disinfected using the above hydrogen peroxide disinfection system. RGP lenses may warp if they are heat-disinfected.
   c. Soft trial fitting lenses can be disinfected using the same hydrogen peroxide system. Some soft lenses have also been approved for heat disinfection.

Other than hydrogen peroxide, the chemical disinfectants used in standard contact lens solutions have not yet been tested for their activity against HTLV-III/LAV. Until other disinfectants are shown to be suitable for disinfecting HTLV-III/LAV, contact lenses used in the eyes of patients suspected or known to be infected with HTLV-III/LAV are most safely handled by hydrogen peroxide disinfection.

The above recommendations are based on data from studies conducted at the National Institutes of Health and CDC on disinfection/inactivation of HTLV-III/LAV virus.[2-4] Additional information regarding general hospital and laboratory precautions have been previously published.[5-9]

Reported by the U.S. Food and Drug Administration; National Institutes of Health; Centers for Disease Control.

Editorial Note: All secretions and excretions of an infected person may contain lymphocytes, host cells for HTLV-III/LAV; therefore, thorough study of these fluids might be expected to sometimes yield this virus. Despite positive cultures from a variety of body fluids of infected persons, however, spread from infected persons to household contacts who have no other identifiable risks for infection has not been documented. Furthermore, there is no evidence to date that HTLV-III/LAV has been transmitted through contact with the tears of infected individuals or through medical instruments used to examine AIDS patients.

References

1. Fujikawa LS, Salahuddin SZ, Palestine AG, et al. Isolation of human T-cell leukemia/lymphotropic virus type III (HTLV-III) from the tears of a patient with acquired immunodeficiency syndrome (AIDS). Lancet (in press).
2. Resnick L, Veren K, Saluhaddin SZ, Markham PD. Personal communication.
3. Martin LS, McDougal JS, Loskoski SL. Disinfection and inactivation of the human T lymphotropic virus type III/lymphadenopathy-associated virus. J Infect Dis 1985; 152:400-3.
4. Spire B, Barre-Sinoussi F, Montagnier L, Chermann JC. Inactivation of a new retrovirus (lymphadenopathy-associated virus) by various agents (chemical disinfectants). Lancet 1984:8408;899-901.
5. CDC. Acquired immune deficiency syndrome (AIDS): precautions for clinical and laboratory staffs. MMWR 1982;31:577-80.
6. CDC. Prevention of acquired immune deficiency syndrome (AIDS): report of inter-agency recommendations. MMWR 1983;32:101-4.
7. CDC. Acquired immunodeficiency syndrome (AIDS): precautions for health-care workers and allied professionals. MMWR 1983;32: 450-1.
8. CDC. Update: prospective evaluation of health-care workers exposed via parenteral or mucous-membrane route to blood or body fluids from patients with acquired immunodeficiency syndrome. MMWR 1985; 34:101-3.
9. CDC. Hepatitis B vaccine: evidence confirming lack of AIDS transmission. MMWR 1984;33:685-7.

Cleaning, Disinfection, and Sterlization of Hospital Equipment

Centers for Disease Control*

Introduction

Cleaning is the physical removal of organic material or soil from objects, and it is usually done by using water with or without detergents. Generally, cleaning is not designed to kill microorganisms but to remove them. Sterilization, on the other hand, has as its goal the complete removal or destruction of all forms of microbial life and is carried out in the hospital with steam under pressure, liquid or gas chemicals, or dry heat. Disinfection describes the intermediate measures between physical cleaning and sterilization and is carried out with pasteurization, ultraviolet radiation, or liquid chemicals. The degree of disinfection accomplished depends upon several factors but principally upon the strength of the agent and the nature of the contamination. Some disinfection procedures are capable of producing sterility if they are continued long enough; when these procedures are continued long enough to kill all but resistant bacterial spores, they are called high-level disinfection processes. Other disinfection procedures kill many viruses and most vegetative bacteria but cannot be relied upon to kill resistant organisms such as tubercle bacillus, spores, or certain viruses; these are called low-level disinfection processes. This guideline deals with the cleaning, disinfection, and sterilization of hospital equipment, a task usually performed by the central services department.

Epidemiology

Parts of the hospital environment can be heavily contaminated with potentially pathogenic organisms, but the objects themselves do not usually cause disease unless they are touched or placed onto the body or unless body fluids flow through them. Thus, contaminated *patient-care* supplies or equipment are the most likely objects of the inanimate environment to cause infection. Ironically, contaminated antiseptics (products designed for use on the skin or other tissue) and low-level disinfectants themselves have also been associated with infections.

---

* Reprinted from the CDC's *Guidelines for Hospital Environmental Control, Part I*, published February, 1981 (revised July, 1982).

Control Measures

Since it is neither necessary nor possible to sterilize all environmental objects, hospital policies should provide for cleaning, disinfection, or sterilization as necessary to decrease the risk of infection. Which process is indicated for an object depends on the object's intended use and, sometimes, the type of contamination. Any microorganisms, including bacterial spores, which come in contact with normally sterile tissue can cause infection. Thus, it is "critical" that all objects which will touch normally sterile tissues be sterile. However, intact mucous membranes are generally resistant to infection by common bacterial spores but not by many other organisms such as viruses and tubercle bacilli; it is "less critical" that objects touching mucous membranes be sterile, although these objects require a disinfection process that kills all but resistant bacterial spores. Intact skin acts as an effective barrier to all but the most virulent organisms, and it is "not critical" that objects which will touch only intact skin be sterile.

Objects potentially contaminated with virulent organisms, such as hepatitis viruses, *Shigella*, or multiply-resistant gram-negative bacilli, may require disinfection even if their use would normally dictate only cleaning. Tubercle bacilli and polio-, coxsackie-, echo-, and rhino-viruses are resistant to most germicidal agents and require high-level disinfection if they are to be reliably eliminated from reusable objects. Bacterial spores are the most resistant and require a sterilization procedure to be reliably eliminated.

Hospitals should perform most cleaning, disinfection, and sterilization of reusable patient-care objects in a central services department to maintain high levels of quality control; in addition, central processing can save money and free patient-care personnel from such activities. However, some hospitals are able to maintain high levels of quality control in closely monitored processing areas other than the central services department, such as an area adjacent to the operating rooms and in the respiratory therapy department.

Reusable objects must be thoroughly cleaned before processing because organic material (e.g., blood and proteins) inactivate disinfectants and protect microorganisms from disinfection and sterilization. Generally, these objects should be cleaned in the central services department. They should not be precleaned in patient-care areas because such precleaning is inefficient and because cleaning by hand can lead to injury and increased exposure to hepatitis virus. However, some objects that are heavily soiled, such as used bed pans, can benefit from precleaning. Before being sent to central services, objects contaminated with infectious materials or objects from patients in certain types of isolation[1] should be wrapped in impervious plastic and marked "contaminated" in order to decrease exposure of personnel to highly infectious microorganisms.

These should be handled with gloves and "decontaminated" before or during cleaning, that is, they should be exposed to a disinfectant or disinfecting procedure to render them safe to handle. Moreover, objects exposed to patients in strict isolation that need to be processed in central services should be decontaminated in the room if they cannot otherwise be safely transported.[1,2]

For many "noncritical" reusable objects in hospitals such as heat lamps, crutches, wheelchairs, bedboards, and bedside utensils, central processing can consist only of 1) high-temperature washing or hand-scrubbing with a detergent or a disinfectant-detergent combination, 2) rinsing, and 3) thorough drying. Many such objects are not easily moved and can be cleaned where they are used. (A discussion of cleaning that is not done in the central services department or other closely monitored areas is included in the Housekeeping Guideline.) Many other objects, including most surgical instruments, can be cleaned by a mechanical washer-sterilizer. However, some delicate instruments might have to be carefully cleaned by hand. Once they are cleaned and inspected, objects requiring sterilization or disinfection are ready for further processing.

Use of pressurized steam in "autoclaves" is the most inexpensive and effective method for sterilization of most objects. Steam sterilization is unsuitable, however, for processing of plastics with low melting points, powders, or anhydrous oils. Residual air pockets can interfere with sterilization in autoclaves; thus, upright containers or steam-impervious wrappers should not be used. After cleaning and before sterilization, objects that will not be used immediately should be wrapped for storage. Sterility can be maintained in storage for various lengths of time depending mainly on the type of wrapping material and the conditions of storage. An item that has been sterilized might not be sterile at the time of use if its safe storage time has been exceeded or if its package has been wet or damaged.

Several methods have been developed to monitor steam sterilization processes, although steam autoclaves are highly reliable if they are used properly. Each sterilizer should be operated according to the manufacturer's instructions. The highest temperature that is reached during sterilization and the length of time that this temperature was maintained should be recorded and checked for adequacy; this check is the most important means of assuring sterility. In addition, heat- and steam-sensitive indicators should be used on the outside of each object. These indicators do not reliably indicate sterility, but they do show that an item has not accidently bypassed a sterilization process. As an additional precaution, a large pack might have an indicator both on the outside and the inside to verify that steam has penetrated the pack. Checks of steam sterilization should be carried out at least once a week using commercial preparations of spores of *Bacillus stearothermophilus* (an organism whose spores are particularly heat resistant, thus assuring a wide margin of safety). If a sterilizer is working properly and used appropriately, the spores are usually killed. A single positive spore test (spores not killed) does not necessarily indicate that objects processed in the same sterilizer are not sterile. It does suggest that the sterilizer should be re-checked for proper temperature, pressure, and use and that the test be repeated. Spore testing should be considered as just one of several methods of assuring adequate processing of inanimate objects in the hospital environment (Table 1).

Implantable objects, for example, implantable orthopedic devices, require special handling before and during sterilization. To guarantee a wide margin of safety, each load of such objects should be sterilized with a spore test, should not be released for use until the spore test is negative (at 48 hours), and should not be sterilized by "flash" steam sterilization (defined as sterilization of an unwrapped object at 270°F or 132°C for 3–5 minutes in a gravity displacement sterilizer). If it is not possible to sterilize an implantable object with a spore test 48 hours before use, then the object should still receive full-cycle steam and not flash sterilization. One acceptable method, steam sterilization at 270°F for 10 min-utes, takes only 5–7 minutes longer than flash sterilization and gives an adequate margin of safety, provided no porous objects (including towels) are included in the load. Packs containing implantable objects need to be clearly labeled so that they can be specially processed.

Because ethylene oxide gas sterilization is a more complex and expensive process than steam sterilization, it is usually restricted to objects that might be damaged by heat or moisture. Before sterilization, objects also need to be cleaned and wrapped. Chemically sensitive indicators should be used with each package to show that it has been exposed to the gas sterilization process. Gas sterilizers should be checked at least once a week with commercial preparations of spores of *Bacillus subtilis* (a resistant spore). All exhaust from gas sterilizers and aerators for gas sterilization should be vented directly to the outdoors be-cause the gas is toxic. All objects processed by gas sterilization need special aeration according to manufacturer's recommendations to remove toxic residues of ethylene oxide.

High-level disinfection can be accomplished by hot-water pasteurization or liquid chemicals. Pasteurization is usually used only for respiratory therapy equipment. Liquid chemical disinfection can be time-consuming and expensive. Several chemical solutions are available (Table 2) for high-level disinfection. Solutions containing activated glutaraldehyde can achieve high-level disinfection in 10 to 30 minutes and sterilization in 10 hours if the objects are cleaned until they are relatively free of organic matter. Gloves should be worn when using chemical disinfectants to prevent skin reactions, especially rashes. A new formu-lation, 6% stabilized hydrogen peroxide, does not appear to cause significant skin rashes and can achieve high-level disinfection in 30 minutes and sterilization in 6 hours. Objects disinfected with liquid chemicals must be rinsed in *sterile* water (or water containing at least 10 mg/liter free residual chlorine, e.g., a fresh 1:5000 dilution of a household bleach that is 5.25% hypochlorite solution) to remove possibly toxic or irritating residues. Afterward, the objects should be handled using sterile gloves and towels and stored in protective wrappers to prevent recontamination.

Recommendations

1. General Operation of the Central Services Department
   a. No disposable object designed for sterile, single use should be resterilized. *Category I*
   b. Any object which should be sterile should not be used if its sterility is seriously questioned, e.g., its package is torn or its expiration date is exceeded. *Category I*
   c. Central services should operate to assure that soiled objects do not contaminate those that are clean. Thus, all contaminated objects should be received and decontaminated in one area and cleaned, disinfected, or sterilized elsewhere. These areas should be separate from those used to receive or store new, clean, or sterile objects. *Category I*

2. Decontamination and Cleaning
   All objects to be disinfected or sterilized should be thoroughly cleaned to remove all blood, tissue, food, and other residue. If necessary, they should be decontaminated before or during cleaning. *Category I*

3. Indications for Sterilization or High-level Disinfection
   a. Patient-care equipment that enters normally sterile tissue or the vascular system, or through which blood flows, should be sterile. *Category I*
   b. Laparoscopes and other scopes that enter the peritoneal cavity should be subjected to a sterilization procedure before each use; if this is not feasible, they should receive high-level disinfection. *Category I*
   c. Endoscopes and respiratory therapy equipment that touch mucous membranes should be subjected to a sterilization procedure before each use; if this is not feasible, they should receive high-level disinfection. *Category I*

4. Methods of Sterilization and Disinfection
   a. Whenever sterilization is required, a steam sterilizer should be used unless the object to be sterilized is damageable by heat, pressure, or moisture or is not otherwise amenable to steam sterilization. *Category I*
   b. Many reusable patient-care objects can be disinfected or sterilized by the methods found in Table 2. *Category II*

5. Method of Processing, Depending on Contamination
   a. Patient-care equipment contaminated with blood from a patient known or suspected to be infected with hepatitis B virus should be sterilized; if this is not feasible, it should receive high-level disinfection. *Category I*

Table 1 Methods of Assuring Adequate Processing of Inanimate Objects in the Hospital Environment

Object Classification	Example	Method	Comment
PATIENT-CARE OBJECTS Sterility is *critical* Sterilized in the hospital: reusable and single use items	Surgical instruments and devices: angiography catheters	Use before maximum safe storage time. Inspect package for integrity and for exposure of sterility indicator before use. Follow manufacturer's instructions for each sterilizer or use recommended protocol. Test sterilizers to find out whether they can kill resistant commercial spores.	Sterilization processes are designed to have a wide margin of safety. If spores are not killed, the sterilizer should be checked for proper use and function; if spore tests remain positive, discontinue use of the sterilizer and have it serviced.
Purchased as sterile	Intravenous fluids; needles; syringes	Use before expiration date if one is given. Inspect package for integrity before use. Culture only if clinical circumstances suggest infection related to use of the item.	Notify the U.S. Food and Drug Administration if factory-related (intrinsic) contamination is suspected.
Sterility is *less critical*, but should be free of most vegetative bacteria Usually disinfected rather than sterilized in the hospital	Respiratory therapy equipment and instruments for gastrointestinal endoscopy that will touch mucous membranes	Sterilize if possible; if not, follow a protocol for high-level liquid chemical disinfection of wet pasteurization. Culture equipment after any important changes in the disinfection process.	These devices come in contact with mucous membranes. Resistant spores can remain after liquid chemical disinfection, but these are not usually pathogenic. Culturing can verify that a disinfection process (or disinfectant) has not resulted in marked increases in recovery of bacteria from equipment.

Purchased	Water, including water for hemodialysis	Use of adequately treated source of hospital water. Store fluids with proper chlorination to avoid microbial proliferation. Perform routine culturing of hemodialysis water.	The risk of disease appears to be related to the number of organisms present (unless virulent organisms are present). Water for hemodialysis may require further processing, e.g., deionization.
Sterility is *not critical* and can be expected to be contaminated with some bacteria	Bedpans; crutches; bed rails; water glasses; linens; food utensils; EKG leads; bedside tables; radiology suites; hemodialysis centers	Follow a protocol for cleaning (use a disinfectant or disinfecting process).	These items will not usually come in contact with open skin or mucous membranes.
NON-PATIENT-CARE OBJECTS[a] Likely to be contaminated with virulent micro-organisms	Laboratories handling patient specimens[b]	Follow a protocol for cleaning (use a disinfectant or disinfecting process).	Areas handling blood or microbiologic specimens are most important.
Unlikely to be contaminated with virulent micro-organisms	Areas not involved in patient care: offices, storage areas	Perform routine cleaning.	Cleaning is aimed mainly at improving the appearance of and providing a proper atmosphere in which to work.

[a] Adequate processing of non-patient-care objects is primarily aimed at protecting personnel and others who come in contact with these objects: sterility is *not critical*.
[b] For disposal of specimens from patients, see Guideline for Hospital Environmental Control: Housekeeping Services and Waste Disposal or *Isolation Techniques for Use in Hospitals* when applicable.

Table 2 Methods of Sterilization and Disinfection

Object	Sterilization — Will enter tissue or vascular system or blood will flow through		Disinfection — High-level — Will come in contact with mucous membranes but not enter tissue or vascular system	Disinfection — Low-level — Will not come in contact with mucous membranes or skin that is not intact
	Procedure	Exposure Time (hr)	Procedure (Exposure Time >10 to 30 min)[a]	Procedure (Exposure Time <10 min)
Smooth, hard-surface	A	mfr. rec.	D	J
	B	mfr. rec.	E	L
	C	10	F	M
	D	18	G	N
	E	6	H	P
			I	
			J	
			Q	
Rubber tubing and catheters[b]	A	mfr. rec.	E	
	B	mfr. rec.	F	
	E	6	H	
			I	
			Q	
Polyethylene tubing and catheters[b,c]	A	mfr. rec.	D	
	B	mfr. rec.	E	
	C	10	F	
	D	18	H	
	E	6	I	
			J	
			Q	

Item				
Lensed instruments	B	mfr. rec.		E
	C	10		Q
	E	6		
Thermometers (oral & rectal)[d]	B	mfr. rec.		K
	C	10		
	D	18		
	E	6		
Hinged instruments	A	mfr. rec.		
	B	mfr. rec.		
	C	10		
	E	6		

Key

A Heat sterilization including steam or hot air (see manufacturer's recommendations)
B Ethylene oxide gas (for time, see manufacturer's recommendations)
C Glutaraldehyde (2%)
D Formaldehyde (8%)-alcohol (70%) solution (corrosion inhibitor needed if formulated in hospital)
E 6% stabilized hydrogen peroxide (will corrode copper, zinc, and brass)
F Wet pasteurization at 75°C for 30 minutes after detergent cleaning
G Sodium hypochlorite (1000 ppm available chlorine) (will corrode metal instruments)
H Phenolic solutions (3% aqueous solution of concentrate)
I Iodophor. Use only a product approved for disinfection by the Environmental Protection Agency (EPA), and follow the product label for use dilution.
J Ethyl or isopropyl alcohol (70%–90%)
K Ethyl alcohol (70%–90%)
L Sodium hypochlorite (100 ppm available chlorine)
M Phenolic germicidal detergent solution
N Iodophor germicidal detergent
P Quaternary ammonium germicidal detergent solution
Q Glutaraldehyde (a 2% solution has been customary for high-level disinfection and has been shown to be effective for high-level disinfection of respiratory therapy tubing by in-use testing. A glutaraldehyde-phenate formulation also has been shown to be effective for high-level disinfection of respiratory therapy tubing at a glutaraldehyde concentration of 0.13%.[3]. Caution should be exercised with all glutaraldehyde formulations when further in-use dilution is anticipated [4]).

Notes

[a] The longer the exposure to a disinfectant, the more likely it is that all bacteria will be eliminated. Ten minutes' exposure may not be adequate to disinfect many objects, especially those that are difficult to clean because they have narrow channels or other areas that can harbor organic material and bacteria.
[b] Tubing must be completely filled for disinfection.
[c] Thermostability should be investigated when indicated.
[d] Do not mix rectal and oral thermometers at any stage of handling or processing.

    b. Most environmental surfaces contaminated with blood from a patient known to be infected with hepatitis B virus should be cleaned with a solution of household bleach (e.g., a 1/10 dilution of a household bleach that is 5.25% hypochlorite solution) because such solutions have good activity against this virus. Hypochlorite can corrode metal and should be rinsed off. Other high-level disinfectants may be used if hypochlorite is not acceptable. *Category II*

    c. Other patient-care and environmental objects that are potentially contaminated with virulent microorganisms should be processed according to the manual *Isolation Techniques for Use in Hospitals*[1]. *Category I*

6. Storage

    Sterile packs should be stored no longer than the safe storage time listed in Table 3. The pack must be considered to be contaminated if the wrap is damaged or has been wet. *Category I*

7. Steam Sterilizers

    a. Steam sterilizers should be monitored at least once a week with commercial preparations of spores of *Bacillus stearothermophilus*. *Category II*

    b. 1) Every load should be monitored with a spore test if it contains implantable objects. These implantable objects should not be used until the spore test is found to be negative (at 48 hours). *Category II*

       2) Implantable objects should not be sterilized by "flash" steam sterilization. *Category I*

Table 3.   Safe Storage Times For Sterile Packs

Wrapping	Duration of Sterility[a]	
	In Closed Cabinet	On Open Shelves
Single-wrapped muslin (two layers)[b]	1 week	2 days
Double-wrapped muslin (each two layers)	7 weeks	3 weeks
Single-wrapped two-way crepe paper (single layer)	At least 8 weeks	3 weeks
Tightly woven untreated pima cotton (single layer) over single-wrapped muslin (two layers)	—	8 weeks
Two-way crepe paper (single layer) over single-wrapped muslin (two layers)	—	10 weeks
Single-wrapped muslin (two layers) sealed in 3 mil polyethylene	—	At least 9 months
Heat-sealed, paper transparent plastic pouches	—	At least 1 year

    [a]Sterility was checked daily for the first week of storage and weekly thereafter.

    [b]Single-wrapped muslin is not recommended because it is easily penetrated by contamination, especially moist contamination.

    Augmented, with permission, from *Hospitals, J.A.H.A.*, by the American Hospital Association, copyright October 16, 1974, Volume 48, no. 20.

8. Ethylene Oxide Sterilizers
   a. Ethylene oxide sterilization should be limited to objects that must be sterilized but can be damaged by heat, pressure, or moisture. *Category I*
   b. Ethylene oxide sterilizers should be monitored at least once a week with commercial preparations of spores of *Bacillus subtilis*. *Category I*
   c. Every load should be monitored if it contains implantable objects. These implantable objects should not be used until the spore test is found to be negative (at 48 hours). *Category II*

9. Dry-Heat Sterilizers
   a. Dry-heat sterilizers should be monitored at least once a month with commercial preparations of spores of *Bacillus subtilis* that are intended to monitor dry heat. *Category II*
   b. Powders and anhydrous oils that must be sterilized should be sterilized by dry heat. *Category II*

10. Positive Spore Tests
    a. If spores are not killed in *routine* spore tests, the sterilizer should immediately be checked for proper use and function; objects, other than implantable objects, do not need to be recalled for a positive spore test unless the sterilizer or its use is defective. *Category II*
    b. If spore tests remain positive after proper use of the sterilizer is documented, its use should be discontinued and it should be serviced. *Category I*

11. Chemical Indicators
    Chemical indicators showing that a package has been through a cycle in a sterilizer should be attached to the outside of each package sterilized. *Category I*

12. Preventive Maintenance
    Equipment used for disinfection or sterilization should be scheduled for preventive maintenance routinely, according to the manufacturers' instructions. *Category I*

References

1. Center for Disease Control. Isolation techniques for use in hospitals. 2nd ed. Washington D.C.: U.S. Government Printing Office. 1975. (DHEW publication no.[CDC] 78-8314).

2. Center for Disease Control. Recommendations for initial management of suspected or confirmed cases of Lassa fever. Morbid Mortal Weekly Rep 1980;28(52suppl):1S–12S.

3. Townsend TR, Wee S, Koblin B. An

efficacy evaluation of a synergized glutaraldehyde-phenate solution in disinfecting respiratory therapy equipment contaminated during patient use. Infection Control 1982;3:240-4.

4. Bageant RA, Marsik FJ, Kellogg VA, Hyler DL, Groschel DHM. In-use testing of four glutaraldehyde disinfectants in the cidematic washer. Respiratory Care 1981;26:1255-61.

Further Reading

American Hospital Association American Society for Hospital Central Service Personnel. Guidelines for the hospital central service department. Chicago: American Hospital Association, 1978.

Block SS, ed. Disinfection, sterilization and preservation. 2nd ed. Philadelphia:Lea and Febiger, 1977.

Center for Disease Control, Decontamination of CPR training mannequins. Morbid Mortal Weekly Rep 1978;27:132,138.

Association for the Advancement of Medical Instrumentation. Good hospital practice: steam sterilization and sterility assurance. Arlington, Va.: Association for the Advancement of Medical Instrumentation, 1980.

Perkins JJ. Principles and methods of sterilization in health sciences. 2nd ed. Springfield, Ill.: Charles C Thomas, 1969.

General Infection Control Guidelines for Pre-hospital Care Personnel

Massachusetts Department of Public Health
Office of Emergency Medical Services

In the pre-hospital care setting, you will probably *not* be aware that a patient is "infected" with the AIDS virus or another communicable disease. Since many potentially infectious persons have no specific symptoms or complaints, they may have no awareness of their potential to transmit their disease to others. Therefore, the following routine precautions should be observed by pre-hospital care personnel for *all* patient contacts:

1. Cover any open cuts or lesions on your own hands with bandages or gloves while rendering patient care. Apply dressings to all wounds on your patient(s) and minimize direct contact with blood or secretions as much as possible. Do not touch your eyes or mouth *before washing your hands thoroughly,* after you have contact with a patient's blood or other secretions.

    If you discover that your patient is infected with the AIDS-associated or hepatitis B viruses *and* is actively bleeding or incontinent; you should wear gloves and gowns to minimize contact with the patient's blood. Wearing a mask is not necessary, since these viruses are spread by blood to blood contact and not via a respiratory route.

2. Always have resuscitation equipment with you to preclude the need for mouth-to-mouth/nose resuscitation. Use of pocket masks by EMT's and First Responders is recommended. Remember the administration of 100% oxygen is preferred and many pocket masks can be connected to oxygen delivery equipment. However, nothing should ever delay the administration of basic life support measures, *i.e.*, CPR.

3. Use extreme caution when removing glass fragments from patients' clothes or body. Use work gloves whenever possible to avoid accidental cuts.

4. Never reapply caps or sheaths to needles or syringes. Cut needle from holder and dispose of all pieces in an impervious container. Do not pass needles from person to person or leave needles exposed at any time.

5. Provide tissues and instruct patients to use them when coughing or sneezing. Wash your hands thoroughly after contact with or disposal of used tissues. If you will be in prolonged contact (1/2 hour or longer) with a patient who is coughing/sneezing frequently, you may wish to wear a mask to minimize your chances of infection.

6. Launder soiled linen, uniforms etc. in hot water and detergent. Use bleach according to directions, whenever possible.

7. Receive appropriate immunizations (rubella, hepatitis B, and tetanus toxoid) and annual tuberculin tests. Establish and maintain communication with the Infection Control Practitioner at each hospital you transport to, for notification of any infectious disease exposures. Be sure to have adequate documentation for every patient contact you have, whether you have transported a patient or not.

8. As indicated in the attached *Cleaning Procedures for Ambulance Equipment and Interior*, clean your vehicle and equipment after *every* patient contact. Be sure to thoroughly clean all equipment used and the interior of the ambulance with an approved disinfectant, in the event of confirmed communicable disease exposure.

Cleaning Procedures for Ambulance Equipment and Interior

Massachusetts Department of Public Health
Office of Emergency Medical Services

Any piece of equipment or surface can become contaminated with any number or type of viruses and/or bacteria, especially those items that come in contact with the victim's mouth, nose or body fluids, *i.e.*, blood. Since many people may be unaware that they are carrying a communicable disease, it is important for EMT's to adhere to a routine cleaning regimen.

After every patient treatment or transport, EMT's should clean up any obviously "dirty" equipment and the ambulance interior to minimize the spread of microorganisms. Any spilled blood must be cleaned up at the first available opportunity. The most important part of the cleaning process is vigorous scrubbing. The friction generated during scrubbing dislodges not only dirt, but also any microorganisms that may be present. For items that are not obviously dirty, a simple washing with hot water and detergent should suffice.

For "hard surface" items, such as the walls and floor of the ambulance, the stretcher, cot mattress, backboards, splints, etc. the EMT should *scrub* these items with hot water and detergent. This should be followed by a scrubbing with a disinfectant, followed by a rinse with clear hot water. Allow surfaces to air dry. (*Note:* wooden backboards and splints must be kept well varnished to prevent water damage and absorption of contaminated fluids).

For "soft surface" items, such as face masks, suction units, bag-valve-mask and demand units, EMT's should check the manufacturer's instructions for the preferred cleaning method.

In general, such items should be scrubbed, while holding them under the surface, in hot water and detergent and then rinsed in hot water. Small brushes may be necessary to clean hard to reach areas.

Next disinfect the items following the manufacturer's specific instructions with respect to the use of alcohol, dilute bleach, or other disinfectants. Some of these products may stain, damage, or be absorbed into some rubber, plastic, or foam products. Alcohol will harden, discolor, and eventually crack most plastic materials. Dilute bleach may corrode certain metals.

Allow items to air dry in order to dissipate fumes prior to use and place them into plastic, self-closing storage bags to protect them from contamination, *i.e.,* face masks, oral/nasal airways, EGTA tubes, bite sticks, laryngoscope blades, etc. EGTA tubes, airways, and bite sticks should be sent for packaging and sterilization after this initial cleaning. (*Note:* items marked disposable must never be reused.)

Note: During the above cleaning steps, EMT's should wear heavy duty rubber gloves to protect their hands from hot water, detergent, etc.

Many hospitals will cooperate with local ambulance services and accept ambulance equipment for sterilization at the hospital. Contact the infection control, central service, sterile supply, or other department that maintains the sterilization equipment. You will be advised as to how the equipment must be prepared and the maximum size that can be fitted into their sterilization device.

In general, equipment must be disassembled, thoroughly cleaned, and packaged in wrappers they may provide. *It is very important to separate* heat and moisture sensitive items from more durable items. Hospitals use a high pressure steam autoclave that sterilizes at very high temperatures (250–280 degrees F). For more sensitive equipment, such as plastics, rubber, and electronic items, an ethylene dioxide gas sterilizer is used. When delivering items to be sterilized, be sure to label these items appropriately so they are not damaged by steam sterilization and do not mix gas and steam sterilizable items in the same packages. Hospital personnel will give you more specific steps to follow.

Oxygen humidifiers (non-disposable) should be cleaned and fresh, distilled sterile water changed at least once a week. Use of plastic, disposable humidifier units is preferred, since each unit may be either transferred with the patient or disposed of after each use.

Linen and uniforms should be laundered in hot water and detergent. When appropriate, use laundry bleach according to directions. (Liquid bleach should not be used on most colored fabrics.)

Helpful hint: Blood stained fabrics can be soaked in hydrogen peroxide and cold water prior to laundering.

Remember, many organisms which have the potential for causing infection can be transmitted to others when emergency care equipment is not properly cleaned. This is especially true of face masks, bag-valve-mask units, demand valve units, and suction units. It is important to completely disassemble and clean these units after each use. EMT's must ensure a safe working environment for themselves and their patients by adhering to a routine cleaning regimen.

These cleaning procedures apply to all cases involving any communicable disease, *i.e.*, AIDS, hepatitis B, tuberculosis, etc. There are no other "special" procedures necessary if the preceding cleaning regimen is adhered to.

Infection Control Guidelines for Handling Blood Products
Visiting Nurse Association of Boston*

Purpose: To prevent acquisition of infection from contact with contaminated blood or items soiled with contaminated blood.

1. Check with physician for the presence of any of the following diseases which require blood precautions:
   a. Hepatitis Viral
      1. Type B (serum, homologous serum hepatitis)
      2. Unspecified type consistent with viral etiology
      3. Hepatitis B antigen carrier
      4. Non-A, non-B

---
* Reprinted by permission. Revised as of April 1985.

b. AIDS

c. Arthropod borne viral diseases: dengue, yellow fever, Colorado tick fever

d. Malaria

e. Creutzfeldt-Jakob disease

2. When working with patients with any of the above diseases, take the following precautions:

a. Hands must be washed before and after each patient contact, following contact with the patient's blood or items soiled with the patient's blood, and as otherwise indicated during patient care.

b. Gloves should be worn when contact with the patient's blood is anticipated.

c. Disposable gowns or disposable protective aprons should be worn when contact with the patient's blood is anticipated.

d. *Special instruments and medical equipment.* No special precautions are necessary *unless* equipment becomes contaminated with the patient's blood.

  • Such contaminated articles should be bagged and disinfected/sterilized before continued use.

e. *Needles and syringes.* Extreme caution must be exercised when handling needles and syringes contaminated with the patient's blood.

  • Always use disposable needles and syringes.

  • Needles *should not* be recapped and should be placed in a rigid, puncture proof container for proper disposal.

It should be noted that all used needles and syringes from any patient should be handled with extreme caution since the possibility exists that a patient's blood may be contaminated with hepatitis virus.

f. *Dressings and tissues.* All dressings, tissues and other disposable items contaminated with the patient's blood must be considered potentially infectious and should be bagged wearing gloves prior to disposal.

g. *Laboratory specimens.* When collecting blood specimens, every effort should be made to prevent contamination of the outside of the collection tube.

  • All blood specimens must be placed in transparent bags and labeled "contaminated" to warn laboratory personnel of potential danger.

Care of AIDS Patient in Home Setting

Visiting Nurse Association of Boston*

AIDS is characterized by variable, often severe suppression of the cellular immune system. The cause of AIDS is unknown, but epidemiological data suggest a transmissable agent, possibly a virus. Transmission of the disease appears to have an epidemiological pattern similar to Hepatitis B and precautions used in Hepatitis B should be used as a guide in implementing infection control procedures. It is suggested that the disease may be transmitted by blood, tissue, secretions, or excretions that may contain blood, *i.e.*, semen, urine, stool, saliva, emesis, and wound drainage. *Meticulous handwashing is necessary.*

Precautions and Requirements	Points to Emphasize
Purpose: to prevent transmission to the organism which can occur from contact with virus.	Transmission of the disease may be via ingestion or inoculation and virus may be present in any secretions. Precautions should be started on admission and maintained throughout length of stay.
Living Space	Strongly recommend own room and bathroom. If common bathroom is used, it should be cleaned with 1:10 dilution of 5.25% sodium hypochlorite solution (household bleach).
Gowns	Should be worn by persons likely to have direct contact with secretions, excretions, or blood.
Masks	Should be worn by workers who have direct or sustained contact with coughing or intubated patients requiring suction.
Gloves	Recommended for persons who are in contact with blood, tissue, body fluids, excretions, or articles/surfaces contaminated by the above.
Syringes/Needles	Dispose in puncture proof, covered container immediately following use. Do not recap, bend, break, or remove needles from syringes.
Personal Care Equipment	Do not share toothbrushes, razors, or enema equipment.
Linen Precautions	Double bag *soiled* linen until ready to wash. Wash separately using hot water and detergent. Dry on "high" in drier.
Dish Precautions	Wash in hot soapy water. Rinse in hot water and air dry. Use dishwasher if available.
Garbage (waste, soiled dressing, tissues, etc.)	Double bag and tie securely.

Reverse isolation may be required in which case gowns, masks, and gloves should be worn by all persons entering the patient's room. Hands should be meticulously washed on entering and leaving the room.

---

* Reprinted by permission. Revised as of February 1986.

Reverse isolation may be required in which case gowns, masks, and gloves should be worn by all persons entering the patient's room. Hands should be meticulously washed on entering and leaving the room.

References

1. *MGH Manual of Nursing Procedures,* Second Edition.
2. Infection Control Guidelines for Patients with the Acquired Immune Deficiency Syndrome (AIDS). *New England Journal of Medicine* 309:740–744, 1983.
3. NYVNS Procedure for Home Care of Patients with AIDS, 8/83.
4. Centers for Disease Control. *Morbidity and Mortality Weekly Report* 34 (November 15, 1985).
5. VNA of San Francisco. "Infection Control Guidelines." *Home Health Care Nurse* (November/December 1984).
6. Shanti AIDS Residence Program. Infection Precautions for Persons Giving Direct Care to Persons with A.I.D.S. in the Home. August 1983.

A Hospitalwide Approach to AIDS

Patricia Navicky, R.N., Infection Control Nurse
Lemuel Shattuck Hospital
Jamaica Plain, Massachusetts

Acquired immunodeficiency syndrome (AIDS) is currently causing considerable concern throughout the United States. This concern is growing more and more every day as the number of cases continues to increase. The impact that this disease is having in all phases of health care delivery is evident. It is because of this that the Infection Control Committee of the Lemuel Shattuck Hospital feels that it is necessary to unify and clarify the approach that we must take in caring for patients with AIDS or possible AIDS.

The following recommendations have been prepared by the Advisory Committee on Infections within Hospitals of the American Hospital Association, with considerable consultative assistance from the Centers for Disease Control and from several hospitals that have had extensive experience with AIDS, and are hereby adopted for use in this hospital.

---

* Reprinted by permission. These policies and procedures are revised as of January 1986. The author would like to thank the members of the Governor's Task Force for AIDS, Department of Public Health, Commonwealth of Massachusetts for their comments and suggestions and also Ira G. Shimp, Chief Executive Officer of the Lemuel Shattuck Hospital, who supported her in promotion of these policies and procedures.

The Definition of AIDS as Applied to Infection Control Measures

The CDC has defined persons for whom precautions should be taken as "persons with: opportunistic infections that are not associated with other underlying immunosuppressive disease or therapy; Kaposi's sarcoma (patients under 60 years of age); chronic generalized lymphadenopathy, unexplained weight loss and/or prolonged unexplained fever in persons who belong to groups with apparently increased risks of AIDS (gay/bisexual men, intravenous drug abusers, hemophiliacs, recipients of blood transfusions, and sexual partners of one of the risk groups); and possible AIDS (hospitalized for evaluation)."

Among opportunistic infections that have been recognized within the AIDS syndrome are pneumonia, meningitis, or encephalitis due to one or more of the following: candidiasis, cryptococcosis, cytomegalovirus, strongyloidiasis, toxoplasmosis, or atypical mycobacteriosis (especially avium-intracellulare species); esophagitis due to candidiasis, cytomegalovirus, or herpes simplex virus; progressive multifocal leukoencephalopathy; chronic enterocolitis (duration of more than 4 weeks) due to cryptosporidiosis; or unusually extensive mucocutaneous herpes simplex (duration of more than 5 weeks).

Included in the definition as of June 1985 are the following individuals:

In the absence of the opportunistic diseases required by the preceding information, any of the following diseases will be considered indicative of AIDS if the patient has a positive serologic or virologic test for HTLV-III/LAV:

a) disseminated histoplasmosis (not confined to lungs or lymph nodes), diagnosed by culture, histology, or antigen detection;

b) isosporiasis, causing chronic diarrhea (over 1 month), diagnosed by histology or stool microscopy;

c) bronchial or pulmonary candidiasis, diagnosed by microscopy or by presence of characteristic white plaques grossly on the bronchial mucosa (not by culture alone);

d) non-Hodgkin's lymphoma of high-grade pathologic type (diffuse, undifferentiated) and of B-cell or unknown immunologic phenotype, diagnosed by biopsy;

e) histologically confirmed Kaposi's sarcoma in patients who are 60 years old or older when diagnosed.

In the absence of the opportunistic diseases required by the current case definition, a histologically confirmed diagnosis of chronic lymphoid interstitial pneumonitis in a child (under 13 years of age) will be considered in26979 tive of AIDS unless test(s) for HTLV-III/LAV are negative.

Patients who have a lymphoreticular malignancy diagnosed more than 3 months after the diagnosis of an opportunistic disease used as a marker for AIDS will no longer be excluded as AIDS cases.

To increase the specificity of the case definition, patients will be excluded as AIDS cases if they have a negative result on testing for serum antibody to HTLV-III/LAV, have no other type of HTLV-III/LAV test with a positive result, and do not have a low number of T-helper lymphocytes or a low ratio of T-helper to T-suppressor lymphocytes. In the absence of test results, patients satisfying all other criteria in the definition will continue to be included.

Confidentiality of the Patient

Because of the publicity that AIDS has received, special care needs to be taken to preserve the dignity and confidentiality of AIDS victims at these times. Incumbent with the need for confidentiality of the patient is the need to ensure appropriate precautions to prevent spread of disease. The procedure that ensures that both the staff and the patient are protected is "BLOOD/BODY FLUID PRECAUTIONS," as recommended in the CDC Guideline for Isolation Precautions in Hospitals. The precautions, but not the diagnosis should be clearly identified. Specimens being sent to the laboratory shall be labeled "BLOOD/BODY FLUID PRECAUTIONS."

Patient Care Precautions

1. A private room is not routinely necessary for the care of HTLV-III/LAV positive patients. A private room is recommended for patients with AIDS who are unable to maintain meticulous hygiene (e.g., those with profuse diarrhea, fecal incontinence, or altered behavior due to central nervous system infections) and these patients should have appropriate supervision when out of the room.

2. To obviate concerns about mouth-to-mouth respiration, portable cardiopulmonary resuscitation equipment, e.g., a disposable ambu-bag with a disposable mask and/or s-tube airway, should be immediately available for use on AIDS patients.

3. Masks are not routinely necessary for the care of AIDS patients. The use of masks is recommended for health care personnel who have direct, sustained contact with a patient who is coughing extensively or a patient who is intubated and being suctioned.

4. The use of gowns is recommended only if soiling of clothing with blood or body fluids is anticipated.

5. The use of nonsterile gloves is recommended if contact with blood or body fluids, secretions, or excretions is anticipated. This recommendation is

particularly important for personnel who have cuts or abrasions on their hands.

6. Hands must be washed routinely when caring for AIDS patients, especially if they are contaminated with blood, body fluids, secretions, or excretions. This precaution should be observed regardless of the use of gloves.

7. The use of protective eyewear, such as goggles, is recommended in situations in which splatter with blood, bloody secretions, or body fluids is possible. This is particularly recommended in the performance of 'rocedures such as endotracheal intubation, bronchoscopy, or GI endoscopy. Precautions during other surgical procedures should be judged on an individual basis.

8. Needles and syringes should be disposable and should be disposed of in rigid, puncture-resistant containers. Needles should not be recapped and should not be purposely bent or broken by hand, since accidental needle puncture may occur. The use of needle-cutting devices is not recommended.

9. Extraordinary care should be taken to avoid accidental wounds from needles or other sharp instruments. Parenteral injections and blood drawing should be planned to keep these procedures at a minimum; they should be carried out by experienced personnel.

10. Blood and other specimens should be labeled prominently with a warning, i.e., "BLOOD/BODY FLUID PRECAUTIONS." The label should accompany the specimen through all phases of processing until ultimate disposal. If the outside of the specimen container is visibly contaminated with blood, it should be cleaned with a disinfectant, such as freshly prepared (once daily) 1:10 dilution of 5.25% sodium hypochlorite (household bleach) with water. All blood specimens should be placed in a second container, such as an impervious bag, for transport.

11. Soiled linens and other laundry should be bagged, appropriately labeled or color-coded, and processed according to the existing policy regarding linens from the patients on isolation precautions. (See section of this manual on "Isolation Techniques" for proper procedure.)

12. Nondisposable articles contaminated with blood or body fluids should be cleaned with a disinfectant, such as freshly prepared (once daily) 1:10 dilution of 5.25% sodium hypochlorite (household bleach) with water before being bagged and labeled and sent to the central supply area for terminal decontamination and reprocessing.

Disposable items should be incinerated or disposed of in accordance with the hospital's policies for disposal of infectious waste. Additional precautions that extend well beyond those currently considered appropriate in light of current knowledge, such as incineration of linens and reusable gowns, or other patient care equipment ordinarily considered reusable, or use of unusual or inappropriate cleaning methods of environmental surfaces, are not only wasteful but contribute further to the unwarranted fear of patients with AIDS.

13. No special precautions for dishes are necessary; either reusable (washed in a dishwasher at 140°F) or disposable dishes may be used.

14. Patients with AIDS who are being transported require no special precautions other than "BLOOD/BODY FLUID PRECAUTIONS." AIDS patients with infections requiring isolation precautions should be managed according to existing hospital policy for Isolation Techniques. Personnel in the area to which the patient is to be taken should be notified of precautions to be used prior to the patients' arrival in that area.

15. Decontamination of surgical equipment, endoscopes, and so forth, should be accomplished by the same sterilization procedures (for such equipment) used for patients with hepatitis B. If possible, surgical procedures on AIDS patients should be scheduled at the end of a day, to allow sterilization of endoscopes overnight (shorter-term procedures result in high level disinfection, rather than sterilization). Invasive patient care equipment should be disposable or must be sterilized. Lensed instruments should be sterilized with ethylene oxide. Ventilator tubing should be either disposable or sterilized before reuse. Instruments that come in contact with blood, secretions, excretions, or tissues, including laryngoscopes, must be sterilized with ethylene oxide before reuse.

16. Blood spills should be cleaned up promptly with a solution of 5.25% sodium hypochlorite, diluted 1:10 water (prepared daily).

17. Routine HTLV-III/LAV screening is currently being considered for dialysis patients. However, until a decision is reached the following is recommended for known HTLV-III/LAV infected patients who may require hemodialysis or peritoneal dialysis. Whenever the possibility of exposure to blood or other body fluids exists it may require the use of gloves alone, as in handling items soiled with blood or equipment contaminated with blood or other body fluids, or may also require gowns, masks, and eye-coverings.

18. Patients with AIDS who must undergo dental procedures should be managed just as patients known to be carriers of HB_sAg. The use of protective eyewear, masks, and nonsterile gloves is recommended if splattering is likely to occur. Dental instruments must, of course, be sterilized after such procedures.

Precautions in Clinical Laboratories

1. The precautions to be taken in clinical laboratories are essentially the same as those recommended for processing specimens from patients known to be carriers of HB_SAg.

2. Mechanical pipetting devices must be used for the manipulation of all liquids in the laboratory. Mouth pipetting must not be allowed.

3. Needles and syringes should be handled as described previously.

4. Laboratory coats, gowns, or uniforms should be worn while working with potentially infectious materials and should be removed before leaving the laboratory.

5. Gloves should be worn when handling blood, tissue specimens, blood soiled items, body fluids, excretions, and secretions, as well as surfaces, materials, and objects contaminated by them.

6. All procedures and manipulations of potentially infectious material is to be performed to minimize the creation of droplets and aerosols. Procedures that have a high potential for creating aerosols or infectious droplets include centrifuging, blending, sonicating, vigorous mixing, and harvesting infected tissues from animals or embryonated eggs. Such procedures should be carried out in biological safety cabinets (class II). Whenever centrifugation of blood or body fluids from AIDS patients is necessary, the use of centrifuge safety cups is recommended.

7. Eating, drinking, and smoking is prohibited in the immediate laboratory area.

8. Laboratory work surfaces should be decontaminated with a disinfectant, such as sodium hypochlorite solution, prepared as previously outlined in item 16 above. This should be prepared on a daily basis and used to wipe up any spills of potentially infectious material.

9. Infectious waste from the laboratory should be processed according to established hospital policy for disposal of infectious waste.

10. Tissue or serum specimens to be stored should be clearly and permanently labeled as potentially hazardous.

11. All personnel should wash their hands following completion of laboratory activities, after removal of protective clothing, and before leaving the laboratory.

12. Pregnant personnel should follow the guidelines recommended in this policy that are outlined in the section entitled "Pregnant Personnel."

Autopsy Precautions

The following recommendations for AIDS autopsy precautions are adapted from joint recommendations of the Centers for Disease Control and the College of American Pathologists and are hereby adopted for use in the Lemuel Shattuck Hospital:

> As part of immediate postmortem care, patients with AIDS or suspect AIDS *should be identified* "infectious hazard (blood/body fluid precautions)" and that identification should remain with the body whether or not an autopsy is carried out, for delivery to morticians.
>
> Double gloves, protective eye covering, masks, cap and gown, and a waterproof apron and shoe coverings should be worn by personnel performing or viewing an autopsy in order to prevent parenteral or mucosal innoculation.

The deceased, and any bagged disposal items, should be tagged as above to prevent unwitting subsequent exposure of other personnel to contaminated articles. Methods that will avoid or minimize aerosol distribution of infectious agents should be used. As an example, bones should be cut with a handsaw rather than an electric saw.

The following should be decontaminated with 0.5 percent sodium hypochlorite at the conclusion of an autopsy:

1. Autopsy table.

2. All contaminated instruments, for 1 hour before washing and autoclaving.

3. Other contaminated items that cannot be disposed of or autoclaved, including the outside of tissue containers.

Tissue samples should be thoroughly fixed in 10 percent buffered formalin before trimming for histology.

Blood and Blood Products

The risk of acquiring AIDS from blood transfusions appears to be very low, on the order of 1:1 million units transfused. Few hospitals or blood banks have the facilities to collect and store blood from directed transfusions for future use or to administratively manage such a program. Autologous blood transfusion is safe in that it does not expose the transfusion recipient to any new diseases or antigens, and such programs should be encouraged (e.g., available through the Red Cross).

There is no evidence, to date, suggesting a possible risk of AIDS associated with the use of immune serum globulin or any of the hyperimmune globulins prepared by generally accepted techniques.

While some pools of Factor VIII concentrate may have contained the putative AIDS agent, the number of hemophiliacs who have developed AIDS is still quite low. Factor VIII concentrate available now has been "heat treated" which has been shown to remove viable HTLV-III/LAV and is thereby now considered safe from AIDS.

Accidental Exposures of Personnel to HTLV-III/LAV

Based upon current information, a significant accidental exposure to AIDS is defined just as is a significant accidental exposure to hepatitis B, that is, accidental parenteral innoculation with blood or blood-contaminated instruments such as needles or other sharp instruments, and mucous membrane or open skin lesion contact with blood or body fluids from AIDS patients. Extraordinary care should, of course, be taken to avoid such accidental exposures. Such accidental exposures do occasionally occur, however, and therefore employees with such exposures should report promptly to the employee health office or to their supervisor.

If a health care worker has a parenteral (e.g. needlestick or cut) or mucous membrane (e.g. splash to the eye or mouth) exposure to blood or other body fluids, the source patient should be assessed clinically and epidemiologically to determine the likelihood of HTLV-III/LAV infection. If the assessment suggests that infection may exist, the patient should be informed of the incident and requested to consent to serologic testing for evidence of HTLV-III/LAV infection. If the source patient has AIDS or other evidence of HTLV-III/LAV infection, declines testing, or has a positive test, the health care worker should be evaluated clinically and serologically for evidence of HTLV-III/LAV infection as soon as possible after the exposure, and, if seronegative, retested after six weeks and on a periodic basis thereafter (e.g., 3, 6, and 12 months following exposure) to determine if transmission has occurred. During tinser this workeriod, especially the first 6–12 weeks, when most infected persons are expected to seroconvert, exposed health care workers should receive counseling about the risk of infection and follow U.S. Public Health Service (PHS) recommendations for preventing transmission of AIDS. If the source patient is seronegative and has no other evidence of HTLV-III/LAV infection, no further follow-up of the health care worker is necessary. If the source patient cannot be identified, decisions regarding appropriate followup should be individualized based on type of exposure and the likelihood that the source patient was infected.

Also, since these patients are often in high-risk groups for hepatitis B, it would seem prudent to follow existing recommendations for hepatitis B prophylaxis. The recommended post-exposure prophylaxis for acute percutaneous exposure to hepatitis B virus is:

Recommendations for Hepatitis B Prophylaxis After Percutaneous Exposure

	Exposed Person	
Source	Unvaccinated	Vaccinated
HBsAg positive	1. One dose of HBIG* immediately. 2. Initiate hepatitis B vaccine series.†	1. Test exposed person for anti-HBs. 2. If inadequate antibody (< 10 sample ratio units by RIA or negative by EIA), give one dose of HBIG* immediately plus hepatitis B vaccine booster dose.
Known source High risk of being HBsAg positive	1. Initiate hepatitis B vaccine series.† 2. Test source for HBsAg; if positive, give one of HBIG* immediately	1. Test source for HBsAg only if exposed person is vaccine nonresponder; if source is HBsAg positive, give one does of HBIG* immediately plus hepatitis B vaccine booster dose.
Low risk of being HBsAg positive	Initiate hepatitis B vaccine series.	Nothing required.
Unknown source	Initiate hepatitis B vaccine series.	Nothing required.

*One dose of hepatitis B vaccine immune globulin (HBIG) is 0.06 mL/kg body weight, intramuscularly. HBsAg = hepatitis B surface antigen; RIA = radioimmunology, EIA = enzyme immunoassay; anti-HBs = antibody to HBsAg.

†Hepatitis B vaccine series is 20 μg intramuscularly for adults, 10 μg intramuscularly for infants or children under 10 years of age. The first dose is given within 1 week of exposure and the second and third doses, 1 and 6 months later, respectively.

No information is available on the potential benefits or problems associated with the use of other active or passive immunizing agents or therapies in this situation.

Public Relations

Public relations issues present both problems and opportunities. Some hospitals have found that the treatment of patients with AIDS has had adverse public relations consequences. On occasion, members of the press have placed disruptive and time-consuming demands upon hospital staff. On other occasions, patients or members of the medical staff have placed inappropriate demands on the hospital, such as by asking that AIDS patients not be treated in the institution. The hospital must not allow these disruptions to interfere with patient care.

In dealing with the press, careful and honest sharing of information will usually diminish adverse publicity, and promote public education. This can be accomplished with the following in mind. First, patient confidentiality and dignity must be preserved. Second, a knowledgeable and authoritative representative of the hospital must designate a representative to the press, and other hospital staff members are required to coordinate all press communications through that representative.

Personnel Management

Some health care personnel, including physicians, have been reluctant to provide hands-on care to AIDS patients. At this time there is no evidence that the risks in doing so are any greater than the risks associated with caring for any other sick persons. The advisory committee recommends that otherwise healthy health care personnel should not be excused on their own request from providing care to patients with AIDS; there is no scientific or ethical reason to do so. If an employee simply refuses to perform his or her duties in relation to caring for AIDS patients, the issue becomes a legal and administrative problem to be resolved on an individual basis. Legal counsel is advised in this situation.

Health care personnel who believe they may be at increased risk because they are immunosuppressed or have other clinical conditionshat mayr that there are certain work assignments that the employee should not accept in relation to the care of AIDS patients, a written recommendation should be provided to the employing department for appropriate action in accordance with the Lemuel Shattuck Hospital's personnel policies and procedures.

Information for Pregnant Personnel

There is no known increased risk to pregnant personnel from caring for AIDS patients. However, many patients with AIDS excrete large amounts of cytomegalovirus (CMV). Both the AIDS virus and CMV are a potential risk to the fetus. Hence, it is recommended that a practical approach to reducing the risk of infection with either the AIDS virus or CMV is to inform pregnant personnel of the potential for teratogenesis. Careful handwashing should of course be stressed after all patient contacts and avoidance of contact with areas or materials that are potentially infective. CMV virus can be shed in the urine, saliva, respiratory secretions, tears, feces, breast milk, semen, and cervical secretions. To date HTLV-III/LAV has been isolated from blood, semen, saliva, tears, breast milk, and urine and is likely to be isolated from some other body fluids, secretions, and excretions, but epidemiologic evidence has implicated only blood and semen transmission.

Personnel with AIDS or Suspect AIDS

To date there is no evidence that health care workers infected with HTLV-III/ LAV have transmitted infection to patients. A risk of transmission of HTLV-III/ LAV infection from health care workers to patients would exist in situations where there is both (1) a high degree of trauma to the patient that would provide a portal of entry for the virus (e.g., during invasive procedures) and (2) access of blood or serous fluid from the infected health care worker to the open tissue of a patient, as could occur if the health care worker sustains a needlestick or scalpel injury during an invasive procedure.

Health care workers known to be infected with HTLV-III/LAV who do not perform invasive procedures need not be restricted from work unless they have evidence of other infection or illness for which any health care worker should be restricted.

Precautions to prevent transmission of HTLV-III/LAV infection from health care workers to patients, regardless of whether they perform invasive procedures are:

1. All HCWs should wear gloves for direct contact with mucous membranes or nonintact skin of all patients.

2. HCWs who have exudative lesions or weeping dermatitis should refrain from all direct patient care and from handling patient-care equipment until the condition resolves.

3. HCWs infected with HTLV-III/LAV should be counseled about the potential risk associated with taking care of patients with transmissable infections and should continue to follow existing hospital policy for infection control to minimize their risk of exposure to othe

Care of AIDS Patients

Precautions are advised for persons and specimens from persons with opportunistic infections that are not associated with underlying immunosuppressive disease or therapy. "BLOOD/BODY FLUID PRECAUTIONS" shall be observed for these categories of patients:

A. Kaposi's sarcoma (patients under 60 years of age)
(patients over 60 years of age who have a positive HTLV-III/LAV antibody titer)

B. Chronic generalized lymphadenopathy, unexplained weight loss, and/or prolonged unexplained fever in persons who belong to groups with apparently increased risks of AIDS:
  1. gay/bisexual males
  2. intravenous drug abusers
  3. blood transfusion recipients
  4. hemophiliacs
  5. heterosexual contacts of persons with HTLV-III/LAV infection

C. Possible AIDS (hospitalized for evaluation) specifically AIDS related complex (ARC)

Patients who merely belong to one of the high-risk groups, but who do not have other clinical evidence of AIDS, do not need these precautions.

It is important to understand that the diagnosis of AIDS in a patient requires only "BLOOD/BODY FLUID PRECAUTIONS," just as for hepatitis B. If a patient with AIDS has another infection or condition requiring additional precautions, then these should be added, according to the *CDC Guideline for Isolation Precautions in Hospitals*. (Also see, Infection Control Manual, LSH, section 22, Isolation Techniques.)

Management of AIDS Patients in the Outpatient Department

The preceding recommendations also apply to the management of patients with AIDS or suspect AIDS in the outpatient clinics of this hospital. Segregated examining rooms for AIDS patients are neither necessary nor desirable. Outpatients with AIDS may use the same waiting areas and bathroom facilities as other patients unless the presence of other infections may require special precautions.

Management of Parenteral and Mucous Membrane Exposure of Patients

If a patient has a parenteral or mucous membrane exposure to blood or other body fluids of a health care worker, the patient should be informed of the incident and the same procedure outlined under the section *accidental exposures* should be followed for both the source health care worker and the potentially exposed patient.

Conclusion

HTLV-III/LAV is transmitted through sexual contact, parenteral exposure to infected blood or blood components, and perinatal transmission from mother to neonate. Patients and workers alike known to be infected with HTLV-III/LAV should not be restricted solely on the basis of this. Specifically, they should not be restricted from using telephones, office equipment, toilets, showers, eating facilities, and water fountains. Equipment contaminated with blood or other body fluids of any patient or health care worker, regardless of HTLV-III/LAV infection status, should be cleaned with soap and water or a detergent. A disinfectant solution or a fresh solution of sodium hypochlorite, (prepared as outlined previously) should be used to wipe the area after cleaning.

References

1. Update on acquired immunodeficiency syndrome (AIDS)—United States, *MMWR* 31:507-14, 1982.

2. Acquired immunodeficiency syndrome (AIDS): Precautions for clinical and laboratory staff. *MMWR* 31:577-80, 1982.

3. An evaluation of the acquired immunodeficiency syndrome (AIDS) reported in health care personnel—United States. *MMWR* 32:358-60, 1983.

4. Update: acquired immunodeficiency syndrome (AIDS)—United States. *MMWR* 32:389-91, 1983

5. Acquired immunodeficiency syndrome (AIDS): Precautions for health care workers and allied professionals. *MMWR* 32:450-51, 1983

6. Update: acquired immunodeficiency syndrome (AIDS)—United States, *MMWR* 32:465-67, 1983.

7. Conte, J.E., Jr., Hadley, W.K., Sande, M. and the University of California San Francisco, Task Force on the Acquired Immunodeficiency Syndrome. Special Report: Infection Control Guidelines for Patients with the acquired immunodeficiency syndrome (AIDS). *New England J Med.* 309:740-44, 1983.

8. Safe Blood for Transfusion. *The Medical Letter on Drugs and Therapeutics* 25:93-95, 1983.

9. Garner, J.S. and Simmons, B.P., CDC Guideline for Isolation Precautions in Hospitals. *Infection Control* 4:326-349, 1983.

10. Summary of recent information: acquired immunodeficiency syndrome. College of American Pathologists, Skokie, IL., July 1983.

11. AIDS case definition revised—Massachusetts Department of Public Health/Boston Department of Health and Hospitals, AIDS Newsletter 1:6, 1985.

12. Recommendations for Protection Against Viral Hepatitis: Recommendation of the immunization practices advisory committee, CDC, department of health and human services; Atlanta, Ga. *Annals of Internal Medicine* 103:391-402, 1985.

13. Summary: recommendations for preventing transmission of infection with HTLV-III/LAV in the workplace. *MMWR* 34:681-694, 1985.

ABOUT THE EDITOR

Michael D. Witt, Pharm.D., J.D. is an attorney at the Boston law firm of Warner and Stackpole. Dr. Witt is an associate editor of *Health Matrix: The Quarterly Journal of Health Services Management*, an interdisciplinary publication of Case Western Reserve University. Also, he serves as a member of the Commonwealth of Massachusetts Department of Public Health Task Force on Needle-Using Drug Abusers and AIDS. Among his other professional activities, he teaches Health and Hospital Law as an Adjunct Assistant Clinical Professor at the Massachusetts College of Pharmacy and Allied Health Sciences.

INDEX

Africa, 166-168
AIDS (Acquired Immune Deficiency Syndrome)
  definition, 4, 29, 195-198, 241-242
  historical aspects, 3-4, 159-163
  patient characteristics, 114
  psychosocial aspects, 58
  societal bias toward, 113
AIDS Action Committee, 92, 127-129
AIDS Medical Foundation, 149-150
AIDS-related complex, 4, 5
  mental health needs, 118
  natural history, 181
AIDS-related virus. See Human T-cell, lymphotropic (leukemia) virus, type III
Ambulance, 100
  cleaning, 235-237
American Hospital Association, 90
  Ethics Committee, 90
American Red Cross Blood Services, 140-144
Antibiotic use, open heart surgery, 54
Antibody testing, 6-7, 95, 135-139. See also Enzyme-linked immunosorbent assay
  abuse, 42
  alternative site, 42, 126, 141
  blood donor, 11-12, 35, 104-105, 126
  confidentiality, 11-12
  decision to seek, 45

health care provider, 12-13, 207-208
hemophilia, 102
historical aspects, 163
military, 46
  report to, 146
necessity, 10-11
positive result, 45, 64, 135-139
prehospital admission, 12-13, 206
premarital, 13, 46
prenatal, 13
purposes, 63
Antidepressant medication, 116
Anxiety, 58
  informed consent, 176-177
Appearance concerns, 114-115
Artificial heart, 54
Assurance of Confidentiality, 104
Autonomy, 14
Autopsy, 219, 245-246
Azidothymidine, 52

Bathhouse, 32-34
  licensure, 33
Behavior modification, 137, 184
  fear, 173-174
Behavioral disease, 32, 162, 169
Beneficence, 154
Bisexual, male, 5, 29
Blood, 7, 140-144
  donor
    altruism of, 140
    vs. recipient benefits, 140-142
    rights, 150-153

screening, 11-12, 35, 104-105
social screening, 142, 147,
149
products, 237-238, 246-247
supply, 140-144
amount, 141
safety, 140-144
transfusion, 5, 8, 29, 142
AIDS risk, 143
non-AIDS risk, 142-143

Burn-out, 125, 129-130

Cancer, historical aspects, 164
Casual contract, 8
Centers for Disease Control, 37-38,
39, 147
certificate of confidentiality, 78-
79
cleaning, 223-233
clinical and laboratory
guidelines, 214-218
disinfection, 223-233
patient guidelines, 195-212
formulation, 212
statistic tabulation, 67
sterilization, 223-233
surveillance, 62
confidentiality, 62
Central nervous system complications, 115
Children with AIDS, 35, 46-47
Cleaning, 223-233
ambulance, 235-237
Clinical trial, double-blind placebo-
controlled, 51-57
historical aspects, 51
historical control, 55-56
subject benefits, 58-59
Cofactor, 64, 65, 135, 170, 180,
181

Common good, 72
Communicable disease, 106-109
defined, 106
Communication, 173-175, 176-177
physician-patient, 174-175
Compassionate plea trial, 54
Competence, defined, 92
Compulsory measures, 8-9
lack of effectiveness, 9
Condom, 63
Confidentiality, 11-12, 36-37, 42,
62-63, 69-71, 74, 91, 97, 182-
183, 188-189, 242
access, 76-78
antibody testing, 11-12
Assurance of Confidentiality,
104
blood bank, 142
certificate of, 62, 78-79, 189
current safeguards, 70
guidelines, 72-86
access, 76-78
activities covered, 73-74
communication, 85-86
continuing advisory board, 85
current legal protection, 78-81
education, 86
formulation, 69-71
identifier, 75-76
information needed, 75
informed consent, 83-84
institutional review board, 81-
83
legal consistency, 84-85
nonresearch access, 77-78
subjects, 74
health insurance, 103
hemophilia, 102
legal aspects, 62-63, 79-81
legislative process, 62-63
physician-patient, 61
military, 61
professional discretion, 70, 80-

81
  voluntary researcher violation,
    67-68
Connecticut Quarantine Statute,
  106-109
Consent, 74
  informed. See Informed
    consent
Contact lenses, trial fittings, 221
Control measure
  historical, 55-56
  legal, 14-19
Cost issues, 38-39, 113, 115, 128
  lost productivity, 128
Counseling, 95

Death, 121-124
  listed vs. real cause, 181
Defense Department Military
    Blood Program, 145-146
Delirium, 115-116
Dementia, 115, 116
Denial, 125-126, 174
Dental care, 99, 101, 219
Dependence, 114
Depression, 58, 115, 116
Diagnosis, 30, 196-198
Diarrhea, 4
Disability, legal aspects, 96-97
Disclosure, deductive, 76
Discrimination
  AIDS patient, 97-99
    litigation, 97-99
  against disabled, 97-98
  homosexuality, 60-62, 65-68,
    89, 95-96
Disinfection, 208-209, 223-233
Donor deferral register, 141, 147
Due process, 16-17
Dying, 121-124

Education, 31, 54-55, 93, 94
  health care provider, 119
Employment, 98-99
Enzyme-linked immunosorbent as-
    say (ELISA), 7, 42, 104, 135.
    See also Antibody testing
  confirmatory, 7
  false-negative, 145, 149
  false-positive, 140, 145, 153
  overinterpretation, 135
  sensitivity, 7
  specificity, 7
  as teaching device, 137-138
Epidemic, secondary social, 3
Epidemic Intelligence Service offi-
    cer, 38
Epidemiology, 5-6, 27, 177-181,
    181-183
  acceleration theory, 6
  saturation theory, 6
Equal protection, 16
Estate planning, 96
Ethical issues, 185-191
Ethical Principles of Psychologists,
    185-186
Europe, 166-167
Eye care, 220-222

Fatigue, 4
Fear, 118-119
  behavior modification, 173-174
Federal government, 38
  research effects, 139
  research risks, 154-155
Fever, 4
Food and Drug Administration, 35
  blood donor screening, 11
Food service worker, 211
Fourteenth Amendment, 15
Freedom of Information Act, 78
Funding, 41, 43-44
  principles, 39

reprogramming, 41-42

Gastrointestinal symptoms, 4
Gay Men's Health Crisis, 127
Geographic distribution, 166-168
    differences, 166-167
Gonorrhea, 159-161
    incidence decrease, 32
Government agency
    intravenous drug user, 67
    record confidentiality, 37
    role definition, 37, 38
Guilt, 114, 116

Haiti, 5, 29, 147
    AIDS introduced to, 28
    epidemiological study, 147-148
Health care provider
    accidental exposure, 247
    AIDS patient death effects, 125
    antibody testing, 12-13
    attitudes, 122-123
    disease exposure, 65
    emergency, 205
    mental health need training, 118
    pregnant, 249
    psychological effects, 65, 66
    refusal to provide care, 249
    support group, 129
    transmission from, 207-208
    transmission to, 203-208
Health department. See Specific
    type
Health insurance, 100-101
    confidentiality, 103
    hemophilia, 102
    informed consent, 103
Helper cell, 4
Hemophilia, 5, 29
    antibody test, 102
    confidentiality, 102

health insurance, 102
    mental health needs, 117
Hepatitis B, 9, 16, 136, 201-202,
    248
    double-blind placebo-controlled
    trial, 53
Herpes simplex encephalitis, 51, 53
Heterosexual partner, 5, 29
Home care, 204-205, 239-240
Homosexual
    attitudes toward health care
    professionals, 60
    discrimination against, 60-62,
    65-68, 89, 95-96
    gay organizations, 31
    illegality of, 61
    life-partner, 96
    legal status, 96-97
    male, 5, 29
    mental health needs, 117-120
    revealed, 114
Hospice, 58
Hospitalization, 122
    antibody testing, 12-13
    patient care guidelines, 195-
    212, 242-243, 250-251
Hotline, 31
Housekeeping, 208-209
HPA-23, 52
Human immunodeficiency virus.
    See Human T-cell
    lymphotropic (leukemia)
    virus type III
Human subject protection regula-
    tions, 154-155
Human T-cell lymphotropic
    (leukemia) virus type III
    (HTLV-III), 4, 29, 44
    biological process, 64
    historical aspects, 40
    mutation, 3
    phenotypic variability, 3
    strain differences, 136-137

transmissability, 7-8

Identifier, 75-76
  precautions, 75-76
  selection, 75
  types, 75
Idoxuridine, 51, 55
Immigration, 167
Immune system, neonatal, 5
Immunofluorescence assay, 7
Incidence, 182
Incubation period, 3, 29
Infant, 5, 6
Infection, AIDS-related, 4
Informed consent, 57-58, 76-77,
    83-84, 91
  anxiety, 176-177
  health insurance, 103
  stress, 176
Insemination, artificial, 138
Institutional Review Board, 57, 81-
    83, 154-155
  risk assessment, 70
Interferon, 56, 57
  bone marrow transplant, 53-54
  side effects, 57
Interferon-alpha, 52
International Conference on AIDS,
    36
Intravenous drug user, 5, 29, 66, 67
  mental health needs, 117
Intrusiveness, 187-188
Isolation
  emotional, 114, 116
  physical. See Quarantine

Jacobson v. Massachusetts, 14
Justice, 154

Kaposi's sarcoma, 4, 30

Kaposi's Sarcoma Foundation, 127
Kenya, 27
Kirk v. Wyman, 15

Laboratory guidelines, 214-218,
    245
Latency period, 3, 29
Least restrictive alternative, 15-16,
    107
Legal aspects
  confidentiality, 62-63, 78-81
  consistency, 84-85
  control measures, 14-19
  discrimination, 96-99
  life-partner, 96-97
  quarantine, 15, 16-17, 18-19
  register, 17-18
  reporting, 17-18
  sodomy, 95
  status as couple, 96-97
  will, 96
Lethargy, 4
Liability, hospital, 12
Life-partner, 121, 126
  status as couple, 96
Litigation, AIDS discrimination,
    97-99
Local health department, 37-38
  role definition, 37
Lymphadenopathy, 4, 5
Lymphadenopathy-associated
    virus. See Human T-cell lym-
    photropic (leukemia), virus
    type III

Massachusetts Department of Pub-
    lic Health, guidelines, 234-
    236
Medical necessity, 15
Military, 66
  blood donation, 146

discrimination against gays, 61
HTLV-III testing, 46
Mortician, 219
Mother, infected, 8
Myalgia, 4

National Institute of Mental Health,
183-184
National Institutes of Health, 39,
154
National Transfusion Safety Study,
105
Natural history, 181
Necropsy, 219
Needle, contaminated, 8, 67
public policy, 67
Neuropsychiatric complications,
115
*New York Association for Retarded
Children v. Carey*, 15-16
Notification, 92-93, 101, 182

Obligation, 89
Office for Protection from Re-
search Risks, 154-155
Origin, 27, 28, 168
monkey, 28
Outpatient care, 251

Pain, 124
muscular, 4
Patient advocate, 92
Patient's Bill of Rights, 90
Patients' rights, 90-93
historical aspects, 90
Peer review, 39, 40
Personal service worker, 210
Phosphonofurmate, 52
Pneumocystis carinii, 4, 30
Pneumonia, 30

Polio, 51
Political conservatism
effect on research, 66, 94
Political controversy
bathhouse closure, 32-34
funding, 41
Precedent, 16
Prehospital care, 234-235
Privacy, 16, 37, 69, 187-189
government records, 37
Privacy Act of 1974, 78
Privilege, 89
Prostitution, 34-35, 66, 163
Psychiatric illness, 113-116, 117-
120
organic basis, 115-116, 118
Psychological research, ethical is-
sues, 185-191
Psychotherapy, 116
Psychotropic medication, 116
Public health, historical aspects,
164-166
Public Health Service, 37
attitude toward gays, 60, 63
resource redirection, 42
Public policy, 8-20, 38, 93-99
classic, 8
intravenous drug user, 67
needle contamination, 67
objective, 8
Public relations, 248
Public service announcement, 31
Public support, 32-34

Quarantine, 93-96, 101
Connecticut statute, 93-94, 101,
106-109
court hearing, 107
least restrictive alternative, 107
legal aspects, 15, 16-17, 18-19
length, 103-104
limited, 18-19

typhoid, 104

Radioactive material, 106-109
Rationality, minimum, 15-16
Register, legal aspects, 17-18
Registry, San Francisco, 30
Regulatory cell, 4
Reporting
  disease vs. carrier status, 17
  legal aspects, 17-18
  San Francisco, 30
Research, 39
  basic vs. applied, 40
  central coordination, 40
  communication, 173
  constraints, 94
  data quality, 66
  double-blind placebo-controlled
    clinical trial, 51-57
    historical aspects, 51
  epidemiological studies, 138-
    139
  ethical issues, 64-65, 67-68, 69-
    72
  ethics, 51-59
  federally funded, 139, 154-155
    confidentiality, 62
  vs. medical care, 73-74
  moral issues, 64-65
  psychological, ethical issues,
    185-191
  vs. public health intervention,
    73-74
  result reporting, 190-191
  risk assessment, 70
  risks, 154-155
  social science, 173-175
  social scientific, 183
  sociomedical, 177-181
  subject benefits, 58-59, 64
  subject trust, 66
  vs. surveillance, 73-74

Resistance, reduced, 199
Respect for persons, 72, 154
Retronrus, 6, 29, 40
Rheumatic fever, corticosteroid for,
  55
Ribavirin, 52
Rights, 89, 93
  blood donor, 150-153
  to care, 99, 100-101
  hospitalized patient, 90-93
    historical aspects, 90
  individual, 60, 90
  societal, 60, 90
Risk, 9
Risk factor, U.S. vs. Africa, 27
Risk group, 3, 5, 29, 95, 200. See
    also Specific type
  constant percentages, 29
  mental health needs, 118-119
  risk gradient, 179-180
Role definition
  government agency, 37, 38
  local health department, 37
  state health department, 37
Rwanda, 27, 166-168

Safe sex, 63, 101-102, 137, 174
Saliva, 7
Scarification, 167
Screening. See Antibody testing
Self-blame, 114
Self-destructive behavior, 174
Self-determination, 14
Self-esteem, decreased, 114, 116,
  118
Self-support network, 129
Semen, 7, 138
Sex club, 32
Sex distribution of AIDS, U.S. vs.
    Africa, 27
Sexual conduct, 8, 101-102, 126
  anonymous, 114

change, 32
exclusivity, 126
heterosexual, 8
homosexual, 8
increased number, 8
receptive anal intercourse, 8
safe. See Safe sex
Side effects
interferon, 57
sudamin, 57
Social disease, 164-166
definition, 164
historical aspects, 164-166
Social service, 116
Social support, 127-130
Sodomy, 95
Sore throat, 4
State health department, role definition, 37
Sterilization, 208-209, 223-233
Stress, 113-116
informed consent, 176
societal, 118-119
Subacute encephalitis. See AIDS
encephalopathy
Subpoena, 70, 80, 81, 103, 104,
142, 189
Suicidal thoughts, 116
Support, 54
Support system, 118
Suramin, 52
side effects, 57
Surveillance, 36
vs. research, 74
Syphilis, 159-161
historical aspects, 44

T-4 lymphocyte, 4
Tears, 7, 220-222
Tranquilizer, 116
Transmission, 7-8, 65, 94, 178-179,
181-182

in Africa, 27-28
cofactor, 64, 65, 135, 170, 180,
181
co-worker, 211
female to male, 8
geographical differences, 166-
167
from health care provider, 207-
208, 249-250
precautions, 207
risk, 207
to health care provider, 203-208
exposures, 205-206
precautions, 203-204
risk, 203
heterosexual, 30
HTLV-III positive vs. symptomatic, 101-102
male to female, 8
nonsexual household contact,
200
prevention
hospital, 195-212, 242-243,
250-251
workplace, 200-202
Transplantation, bone marrow, interferon, 53-54
Treatment, right to refuse, 91-92
Trial. See Clinical trial and Compassionate plea trial
Trust, 68, 142
Tuberculosis, 164, 165

Unemployment, 115

Vaginal secretions, 7
Venereal disease, 159-163
Virus. See Specific type
Visiting Nurse Association of
Boston, guidelines, 237-240
Voluntary measures, 9, 14

Ward, for AIDS cases, 31
Waste disposal, 208-209
Western blot analysis, 7, 153
Will, 96

Zaire, 27, 166-168